UR
REN

The Authors

J. E. NEWSAM
M.B., Ch.B., F.R.C.S. (Edin.),

Consultant Urological Surgeon,
Western General Hospital, Edinburgh.

J. J. B. PETRIE
B.Sc., M.B., Ch.B., M.R.C.P.

Senior Medical Registrar,
Renal Unit, Royal Infirmary, Edinburgh.

Urology and Renal Medicine

J. E. NEWSAM
J. J. B. PETRIE

E & S LIVINGSTONE
EDINBURGH AND LONDON
1971

ISBN 0 443 00763 2

Printed in Great Britain

PREFACE

This book is intended primarily for undergraduates and presents a brief account of surgical and medical disorders of the kidneys and of the urinary and male genital tracts. It is considered that there are many advantages in a combined text of this kind, because to divide a subject into medical and surgical compartments is artificial and is apt to result in the duplication of some topics and the neglect of others. Controversy is an integral part of medicine but in a book of this size it is not possible to weigh opposing views impartially and presentation is of necessity somewhat dogmatic. However, for those whose interest is stimulated to further study, more detailed and lengthier books are suggested at the end of each chapter.

1971

J. E. NEWSAM
J. J. B. PETRIE

CONTENTS

Chapter 1

THE STRUCTURE AND FUNCTION OF THE KIDNEYS

The excretion of waste products is the most obvious function of the kidneys, but to regard them solely, or even primarily, as organs of excretion is a mistake. If cells are to function normally they must have a constant internal environment. The kidneys are largely responsible for controlling the volume, osmotic concentration and electrolyte content of this environment. They also have endocrine functions which are concerned with the regulation of blood pressure and the control of red cell production. It is not surprising that disordered renal function can affect almost every system in the body.

A clear understanding of the structure and function of the kidneys is essential for the diagnosis and management of renal disorders.

THE STRUCTURE OF THE KIDNEYS

The kidneys are paired organs which lie on the posterior abdominal wall behind the peritoneum. Each kidney is about 12 cm in length and weighs about 150 g. The centre of the medial aspect of the kidney is concave and occupied by a deep fissure called the hilum, which transmits the renal vessels and nerves and which contains the renal pelvis. The kidney is composed of an internal medulla and an external cortex. The medulla consists of the renal pyramids, the bases of which are directed towards the cortex, while the apices converge and project into the calyces as the renal papillae (Fig. 1).

The functional unit of the kidney is the nephron, which consists of a glomerulus and a renal tubule. The glomerulus is a network of capillaries fed by a relatively wide-bore afferent arteriole, and drained by a somewhat narrower efferent arteriole. The two arterioles are in close proximity to each other and form

1

what is sometimes called the 'stalk' of the glomerulus.

The entire glomerulus apart from the stalk is invested in a capsule, called Bowman's capsule, which is the invaginated blind proximal end of the renal tubule, and which has two layers, a

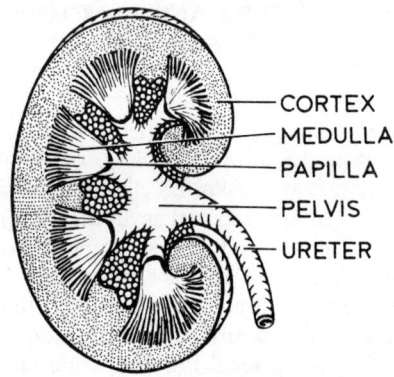

Fig. 1. Gross structure of the kidney.

visceral and a parietal. The glomerular filter is made up of three layers. The innermost consists of the cells of the capillary itself and is called the endothelial cell layer. The outer is the visceral layer of Bowman's capsule, and called the epithelial cell layer. The third layer lies between the endothelial and epithelial cells and is called the basement membrane (Fig. 2).

Spaces known as slit pores exist in both the endothelial and the epithelial cell layers, and have a diameter of 100 to 200 Å. Since the glomerulus is virtually impermeable to molecules with a diameter of over 60 Å, the main barrier to filtration is not the slit pores but the basement membrane.

For descriptive purposes the renal tubule is divided into four parts (Fig. 3). The first part is tortuous and is known as the proximal convoluted tubule. Its luminal border is called a 'brush border' because it has numerous narrow and deep indentations which provide a large surface area. The cells are cuboidal, and contain many mitochondriae — a fact that suggests intense enzymatic activity. Structurally the proximal convoluted tubule is well suited to active reabsorption and reabsorbs no less than four-fifths of the glomerular filtrate.

The second part of the tubule is called the loop of Henle. It

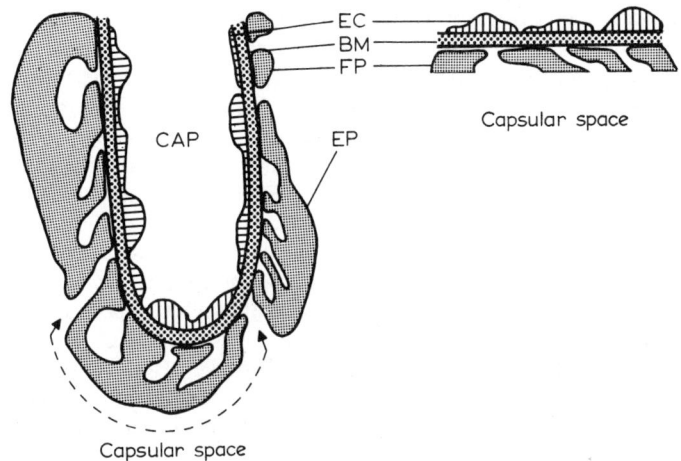

Fig. 2. The glomerular filter as seen on electron microscopy. CAP – capillary lumen; EC – endothelial cell layer; BM – capillary basement membrane; EP – epithelial cell layer; FP – foot processes of the epithelial cells.

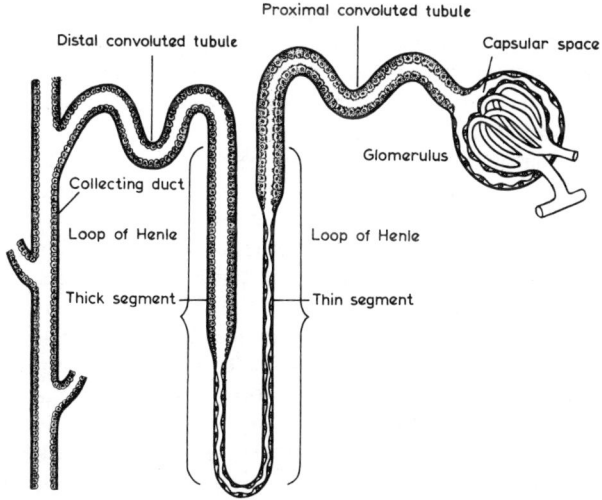

Fig. 3. The nephron.

3

descends into the renal medulla, bends sharply and ascends to re-enter the cortex. The descending limb of the loop, the bend, and the proximal part of the ascending limb are all lined by flat epithelium, whereas the distal part of the ascending limb is lined by cuboidal cells. The loop of Henle plays an essential part in the concentration of urine and the longer it is the more concentrated can urine be made. The kangaroo rat, which lives in the desert and which is able to survive for months on the water derived from the metabolism of dry grain, has the longest loops of Henle in proportion to its size in the animal kingdom, and produces urine which is three times as concentrated as that which man can produce even in his most dehydrated state.

The third part of the tubule is called the distal convoluted tubule, and lies, like the first part, in the cortex. Its cuboidal cells have fewer mitochondriae than those of the proximal tubule, and do not possess brush borders.

The fourth part of the tubule is called the collecting duct. Each collecting duct runs a fairly straight course through the renal medulla, uniting with other collecting ducts en route. The relatively large final channels are known as the ducts of Bellini. These run to the tips of the renal papillae, where they open into the renal calyces.

Developmentally, the collecting ducts arise from the ureteric buds. At one time they were regarded as simple conduits which played little part in the modification of the glomerular filtrate. It is now known, however, that the collecting ducts have an important role in the final adjustment of the volume, acidity and salt content of the urine.

In mammals the tubules receive their blood supply through a peritubular complex of capillaries which arises from the efferent arteriole. The blood reaching the tubular capillaries has already passed through the glomerular capillaries of the same nephron. Thus the kidneys, like the liver and the pituitary, have a portal circulation.

In addition to a peritubular capillary plexus, the efferent arterioles draining the glomeruli situated nearest to the medulla give rise to capillary sized vessels known as the vasa recta. These descend into the medulla, bend sharply and re-ascend into the cortex, where they drain into venules. The vasa recta are concerned, along with the loops of Henle and the collecting ducts, with the concentration of the urine.

Production of the Glomerular Filtrate

Man and most other animals produce urine primarily by glomerular filtration. The volume and the composition of the glomerular filtrate, however, is considerably modified by the tubules (see Fig. 9).

Since there is little vascular resistance between the aorta and the wide-bore afferent arterioles, the pressure in the glomerular capillaries is high. The efferent arterioles are narrower than the afferent vessels. The glomerular capillaries are thin-walled, and have a large surface area. All these factors combine to produce a system ideally suited to high pressure ultrafiltration.

The amount of glomerular filtrate is determined by the filtration force at the glomeruli and by the number of functioning glomeruli. The filtration force is the hydrostatic pressure at the glomerulus (about 60 mm Hg) minus the osmotic pressure of the plasma proteins (25 mm Hg) and the back pressure in the capsular space (about 10 mm Hg). The glomerular filtration rate is normally about 120 ml per minute, or 170 litres per 24 hours.

Complex nervous and humoral mechanisms control renal blood flow but, in general, lowering the renal artery pressure reduces the filtration rate. Reducing the concentration of plasma proteins or the back pressure in the capsular space increases the glomerular filtration rate, while increasing them reduces it.

In 1924 Richards and his colleagues introduced a technique for sampling the fluid in the capsular space and tubules of the frog with micro-pipettes; later the technique was used on mammalian kidneys. Analysis of fluid obtained from Bowman's capsule has shown it to be an ultrafiltrate of plasma. Its composition with respect to small molecular weight substances is almost identical to that of plasma, but it contains only about 20 mg per cent of protein — a concentration less than 0.5 per cent of the 7.0 g protein/100 ml which is present in plasma.

Renal Clearance

The renal clearance of a substance can be defined as the number of millilitres of plasma which contain the amount of the substance excreted in the urine in one minute.

Renal clearances can be used to measure glomerular filtration rate and renal blood flow, and also to study the behaviour of substances as they pass through the renal tubules. The renal clearance of any substance can be determined as follows. A timed specimen of urine is collected and a sample of blood is taken near the mid-point of the collection period. The volume of urine is measured, and the concentration of the substance concerned is determined in both plasma and urine. (Confusion is avoided if both concentrations are expressed as mg per ml.)

If U is the concentration of the substance in the urine, in mg/ml,

V is the volume of the urine collection (in ml),

T is the duration of the collection period (in minutes),

then the amount of the substance excreted in the urine in one minute is

$$\frac{UV}{T} \text{ mg}$$

If the plasma concentration of the substance is P, the *volume of plasma* which *contains the amount of the substance excreted in one minute* is

$$\frac{UV}{PT} \text{ ml}$$

This is the renal clearance.

Determination of glomerular filtration rate

Homer Smith found in dogs that inulin, creatinine, ferrocyanide, thiosulphate and mannitol all had the same renal clearance. This clearance was unaltered by varying the plasma concentrations of the substances concerned. He thought it unlikely that the chemical processes of tubular reabsorption and tubular secretion could proceed at precisely the same rate for such different substances, and postulated that they were all excreted solely by glomerular filtration, and were neither secreted nor reabsorbed in the tubules. It follows that the volume of plasma 'cleared' of inulin or endogenous creatinine is the volume of plasma filtered at the glomeruli, and that the clearance of inulin or endogenous creatinine measures the glomerular filtration rate. (In man some endogenous creatinine is secreted by the renal tubules, and the clearance of creatinine is slightly higher than the glomerular filtration rate.)

6

Tubular Reabsorption and Tubular Secretion

Some substances are reabsorbed from the tubular lumen. Others are secreted into it by the tubular cells. Figures 4 and 5 show the relationship which exists between plasma concentration and urinary excretion, and between plasma concentration and renal clearance, for substances handled by the tubules in different ways.

In Figure 4, line 1 represents a substance, such as inulin, which

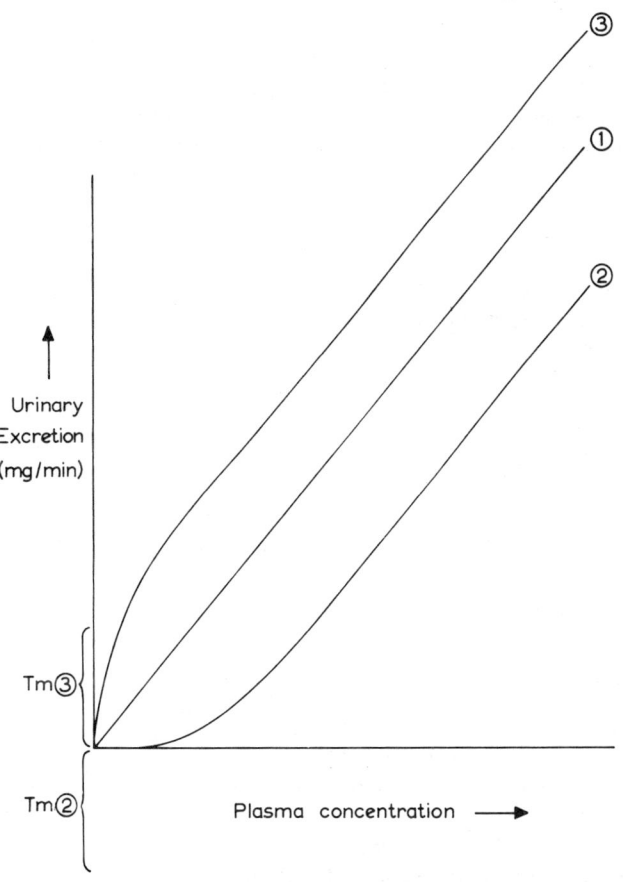

Fig. 4. Urinary excretion at various plasma levels of substances handled in different ways by the renal tubules. (For explanation see text.)

is filtered at the glomeruli but neither reabsorbed nor secreted by the tubules. What is filtered is excreted, and excretion is therefore directly proportional to plasma concentration.

Line 2 represents a substance which (like glucose) is filtered and reabsorbed, but which is not secreted. At low plasma concentrations all that is filtered is reabsorbed, and none of the substance appears in the urine. Active reabsorption proceeds at a finite rate, however, and there is a limit to its extent. When the amount of the substance filtered at the glomeruli becomes greater than the tubular reabsorptive capacity, the substance appears in the urine. The plasma level at which this occurs is known as the renal threshold for the substance concerned. Once reabsorption is fully saturated, any further increase in plasma concentration results in a corresponding increase in urinary excretion. Line 2 becomes parallel to line 1, and the vertical distance between the two lines is a measure of the tubular reabsorptive capacity of the kidneys for substance 2.

Line 3 in Figure 4 represents a substance which is filtered and secreted, but which is not reabsorbed. At low plasma levels, excretion rises steeply with plasma concentration. Once the tubular secretory capacity has been saturated, however, any further increase in excretion with rising plasma levels is due entirely to the increase in the amount of substance 3 filtered at the glomeruli. Line 3 becomes parallel to line 1, and lies above it by an amount which is a measure of the tubular secretory capacity for substance 3.

From Figure 5 it can be seen that the renal clearance of a substance which is neither reabsorbed nor secreted (line 1) is constant, regardless of plasma level. This clearance is equal to the glomerular filtration rate. For substances which are reabsorbed by the tubules, but not secreted (line 2), the clearance is zero at low plasma levels, but rises to approach the glomerular filtration rate at high plasma concentrations. For substances which are secreted but not reabsorbed (line 3) the clearance at low plasma concentrations is higher than the glomerular filtration rate, but at high plasma concentrations, the clearance falls, and line 3 approaches line 1.

Para-amino hippuric acid (PAH) and the measurement of renal plasma flow

Para-amino hippuric acid is actively secreted by the renal

tubular cells. Blood samples taken from the renal artery and renal vein show that only 5 per cent of the PAH which enters the kidney leaves in the renal venous blood. The remaining 95 per cent is excreted in the urine.

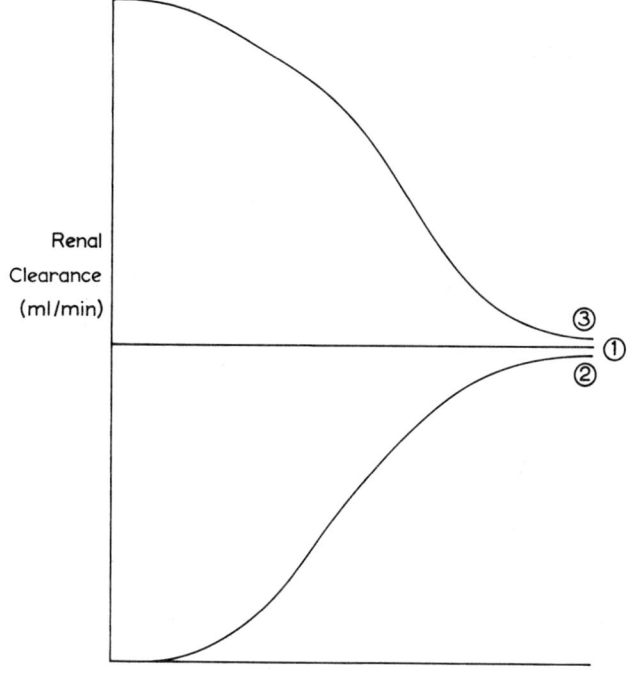

Fig. 5. Renal clearance at various plasma levels of substances handled in different ways by the renal tubules. (For explanation see text.)

PAH can be used to measure renal plasma flow, using the Fick principle; that is to say, if we know how much PAH leaves the kidney in the urine per minute, and the fall in PAH concentration between renal arterial plasma and renal venous plasma, we can calculate the amount of plasma which has flowed through the kidney.

If U is the concentration of PAH in the urine (mg/ml),

V the volume of urine collected (ml), and

T the duration of the collection period (min),

9

the amount of PAH excreted in one minute in the urine is $\dfrac{UV}{T}$ (mg). If Pa is the concentration of PAH in the renal artery, Pv the concentration in the vein, both in mg/ml, $(Pa - Pv)$ represents the amount of PAH lost in the urine by 1 ml of plasma. The amount in the urine, $\dfrac{UV}{T}$, must therefore have been lost by $\dfrac{UV}{T(Pa - Pv)}$ ml of plasma, which is the amount of plasma flowing through the kidney in one minute. If we ignore the small amount of PAH which remains in the renal vein, this becomes $\dfrac{UV}{PaT}$. With a constant slow infusion of PAH the concentration of PAH in the renal artery (Pa) is the same as that in a *peripheral* vein, and renal plasma flow can then be regarded as $\dfrac{UV}{PT}$ which is the clearance value of PAH. The renal clearance of PAH is thus a measure of renal plasma flow, provided the plasma concentration of PAH is sufficiently low.

Renal Handling of Sodium

Sodium is freely filtered at the glomeruli and actively reabsorbed by the tubules. Under normal circumstances, about 1 per cent of the filtered sodium appears in the urine; 7,000 mEq are filtered daily, and 70 mEq are excreted. Under conditions of salt deprivation, however, the urine can become virtually sodium free, with a 24-hour excretion of 5 mEq or less.

Four-fifths of the filtered sodium is reabsorbed in the proximal convoluted tubule. As positively charged sodium ions leave the tubular lumen, negatively charged chloride ions must follow, for reasons of electrical neutrality. The loss of sodium and chloride from the tubular fluid leaves it osmotically dilute and, as a result, water diffuses out of the tubule into the blood stream. Because of the active reabsorption of 80 per cent of the filtered sodium in the proximal tubule, 80 per cent of the filtered chloride and 80 per cent of the filtered water are reabsorbed in this part of the nephron.

Most of the sodium which reaches the distal tubule is reabsorbed by an ion exchange mechanism. The positively charged sodium ions are not simply removed from the tubular lumen — they are replaced by positively charged potassium and

10

hydrogen ions (Fig. 6). The ion exchange mechanism is potentiated by the hormone aldosterone, derived from the adrenal cortex. In the absence of aldosterone, a little over 2 per cent of the filtered sodium escapes into the urine. In the presence of maximal aldosterone activity, the urine becomes almost sodium-free. Because of the large amount of sodium filtered in 24 hours (the total amount of sodium present in the body passes into the glomerular filtrate about five times a day) very small

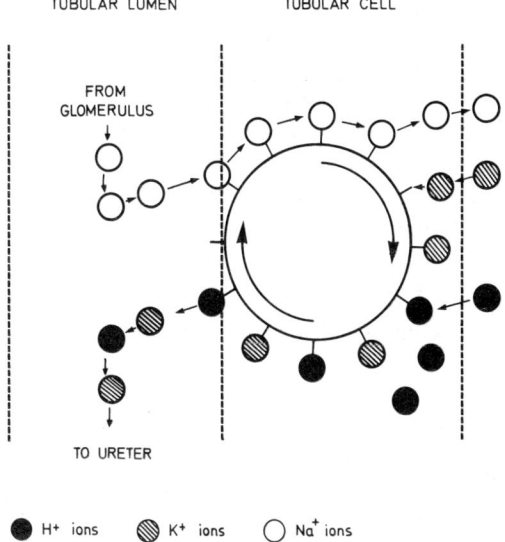

TUBULAR LUMEN TUBULAR CELL TISSUE FLUID

FROM GLOMERULUS

TO URETER

● H^+ ions   ▨ K^+ ions   ○ Na^+ ions

Fig. 6. Tubular reabsorption of sodium ions in exchange for potassium or hydrogen ions.

adjustments to sodium in terms of the percentage reabsorbed have large effects in terms of the body's content of sodium.

The *osmotic concentration* of the body fluids is determined by the anti-diuretic hormone of the posterior pituitary. Provided that there is free access to water, the *volume of the extracellular fluid* is determined by the sodium content of the body, and this is regulated by the kidneys. Salt depletion has profound effects on plasma volume, cardiac output and blood pressure. It is perhaps hardly surprising that among the many homeostatic functions of the kidneys, preservation of sodium balance appears to take

11

precedence. An example of this is seen in the protracted vomiting of pyloric stenosis. The vomitus contains a considerable amount of hydrogen ions, and a moderate amount of sodium and potassium. There is a stimulus to conserve sodium, potassium and hydrogen ions, but in severe cases the drive to conserve sodium over-rides other considerations. Under the influence of aldosterone, sodium is avariciously reabsorbed in exchange for potassium and hydrogen ions, and we get the paradox of a severely alkalotic, potassium-depleted patient passing an acid urine which is rich in potassium.

The Renal Handling of Potassium

Potassium is freely filtered at the glomeruli. Under normal circumstances about 5 per cent of the filtered load is excreted — a fact which indicates considerable tubular reabsorption. In some patients with renal failure, however, the clearance of potassium is greater than the clearance of inulin. In this situation, since the amount excreted is more than the amount filtered, tubular secretion of potassium is obviously present.

From experiments involving micropuncture of the nephron at various sites, we now know that practically all the filtered potassium is reabsorbed in the proximal part of the nephron. The potassium which appears in the urine is derived from tubular secretion in the distal tubule and collecting ducts. This secretion is by way of the ion exchange mechanism for sodium reabsorption.

When diuretics block sodium reabsorption in the proximal nephron, a large amount of sodium is delivered to the distal nephron. Much of this is reabsorbed by ion exchange, and urinary potassium loss is high. Because of the potassium loss induced by diuretics, it is usually necessary to give a potassium supplement to patients who are receiving them.

The Renal Regulation of Acid-Base Balance

If cells are to function normally, the pH of the extracellular fluid must be maintained between 7.35 and 7.45.

The first line of defence against a change in pH is the blood buffering system. The principal buffer in the blood is the bicarbonate/carbonic acid system. The blood pH is given by the Henderson-Hasselbach equation

12

$$pH = pK + \log \frac{\text{Bicarbonate}}{\text{Carbonic Acid}}$$

where pK is the dissociation constant of carbonic acid.

Most of the acid derived from metabolism results from the production of carbon dioxide in the tissues. This combines with water to give carbonic acid; in the lungs carbonic acid dissociates, and the CO_2 produced is eliminated in the expired air.

About 60 mEq daily of acids other than carbonic acid are also produced. Since these acids cannot be eliminated by the lungs, they are called 'fixed acids'. The hydrogen ions derived from fixed acids are buffered by bicarbonate ions.

$$H^+A' + Na^+HCO_3' \rightarrow H_2CO_3 + Na^+A'$$

The carbonic acid produced dissociates and the resultant carbon dioxide is eliminated in the lungs; hydrogen ions are buffered effectively, but bicarbonate is used up in the process. If the body is to be protected against wild swings in pH, the bicarbonate used up in buffering fixed acids must be regenerated.

The role of the kidneys in combating acidosis lies in the regeneration of the bicarbonate used up in neutralizing 'fixed acid' (Fig. 7). This role is carried out by the secretion of hydrogen ions into the tubular lumen. This process leads (directly or indirectly) to:

1. Reabsorption of filtered bicarbonate.
2. Lowering of the pH of the tubular fluid.
3. The excretion of titratable acid.
4. The manufacture and secretion of ammonia (Fig. 8).

The tubular reabsorption of bicarbonate

If the bicarbonate filtered at the glomeruli is allowed to escape into the urine, the blood buffers will become depleted. The kidneys not only have to replace the bicarbonate lost from the body in buffering fixed acids, but have to hold on to the bicarbonate already present in the circulation. Since cells are relatively impermeable to bicarbonate, it is reabsorbed in a rather roundabout way.

Carbon dioxide and water combine in the tubular cell to give carbonic acid. This reaction is accelerated by the enzyme carbonic anhydrase. The carbonic acid dissociates to give hydrogen ions and bicarbonate ions. The hydrogen ions pass into the

13

tubular lumen, where they combine with the bicarbonate present in the glomerular filtrate to give carbonic acid. The hydrogen ions entering the tubular lumen are exchanged for sodium ions, and these sodium ions pass into the blood stream along with the bicarbonate produced in the tubular cells. The carbonic acid produced in the tubular lumen from the secreted hydrogen ions and the filtered bicarbonate ions dissociates to water and carbon dioxide. Both these substances diffuse out of the tubular lumen, into the tubular cell. Here carbonic anhydrase acts to produce carbonic acid once again, and the cycle is repeated (Fig. 8A).

The lowering of the urinary pH

Once all the bicarbonate in the tubular lumen has been reabsorbed, further secretion of hydrogen ion leads to a fall in the pH of the tubular fluid. This fall in pH occurs in the distal tubule

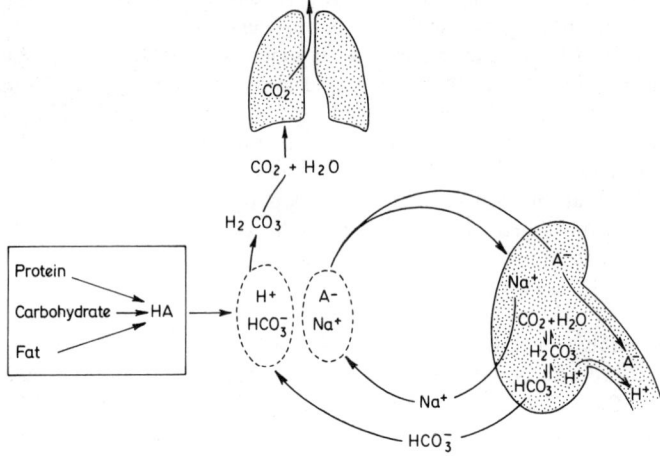

Fig. 7. The role of the kidneys and the lungs in maintaining acid-base balance.

$$pH = pK + Log \frac{\text{Bicarbonate concentration}}{\text{Carbonic acid concentration}}$$

The kidneys regenerate the bicarbonate which is used up when acid is buffered in the blood stream. The lungs eliminate the carbonic acid which is produced when acid is buffered. In crude terms, therefore

$$pH \text{ is determined by } \frac{\text{Kidneys}}{\text{Lungs}}$$

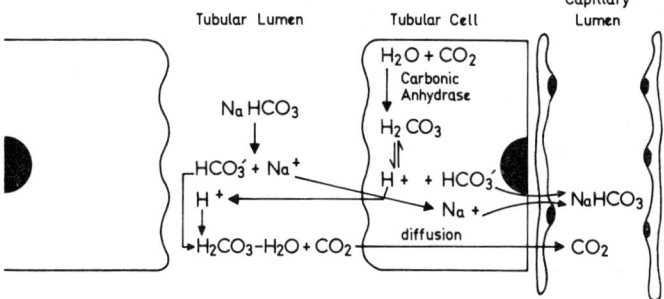

A. Reabsorption of bicarbonate.

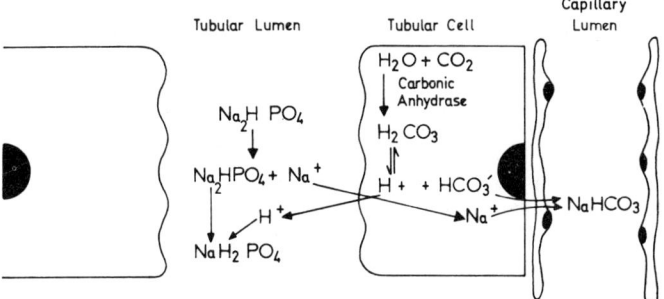

B. Formation of titratable acid.

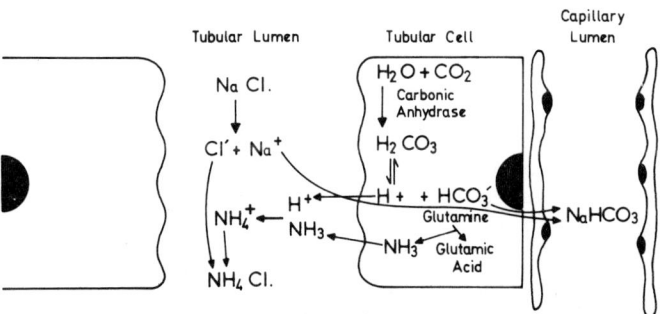

C. Excretion of ammonia.

Fig. 8. Mechanisms involved in the excretion of hydrogen ions by the kidneys.

15

and collecting duct. In acidosis, a pH of 7.4 at the glomerulus can fall to 4.5 in the collecting duct (a hydrogen ion concentration in urine which is 800 times that in plasma).

Excretion of titratable acid

The addition of very small amounts of hydrogen ion to distilled water leads to a marked fall in pH. The presence of buffers in the tubular fluid, however, permits the addition of large amounts of hydrogen ion for a moderate pH change. The main urinary buffer is phosphate.

$$Na_2 HPO_4 + H^+Cl' \rightarrow Na H_2 PO_4 + Na^+Cl'$$

Phosphate is an inefficient buffer at pH 7.4, but is very effective at the hydrogen ion concentration of tubular fluid. Urinary buffers converted to their acid forms are excreted in the urine as 'titratable acid' (Fig. 8B).

The excretion of ammonia

The distal tubular cells contain the enzyme glutaminase, which splits glutamine into glutamic acid and ammonia (Fig. 8C). Ammonia is extremely diffusible, and passes readily into the tubular lumen, where it combines with hydrogen ions to form positively charged ammonium ions:

$$NH_3 + H^+Cl' \rightarrow NH_4^+ + Cl'$$

If there are large numbers of hydrogen ions in the tubular lumen, the conversion of ammonia to the ammonium ion will proceed rapidly. The elimination of ammonia on the tubular side of the cell wall speeds up diffusion of ammonia out of the cell, and removal of ammonia from the cell speeds up the production of further ammonia. More ammonia is therefore secreted into an acid than into an alkaline urine.

The conversion of ammonia to ammonium ions removes hydrogen ions from solution, but the hydrogen ions concerned are none the less eliminated from the body. This mechanism allows the excretion of large amounts of hydrogen ion without an undue lowering of urinary pH. If it is remembered that the urine pH cannot fall below 4.5, it will be apparent that a mechanism which can remove acid from the body without lowering the urine pH significantly is valuable in eliminating an acid load.

The Kidneys and Water Balance

170 litres of water are filtered daily, but only about 1.5 litres of urine are produced in 24 hours. Over 168 litres of water are therefore reabsorbed by the renal tubules.

Since the proximal convoluted tubule is freely permeable to water, no osmotic gradient can exist between it and the blood perfusing the renal cortex. The active reabsorption of 80 per cent of the filtered sodium (along with 80 per cent of the filtered chloride) results in the passive diffusion of 80 per cent of the filtered water out of the proximal tubular lumen.

The proportion of the glomerular filtrate which is reabsorbed in the distal parts of the nephron is more variable. If dehydration is present the urine flow may fall to less than 0.5 ml per minute. If, on the other hand, there is an excess amount of water in the body a water diuresis will result. Almost all the water which reaches the distal nephron may pass into the urine, and the urine flow may approach 20 ml per minute (Fig. 9).

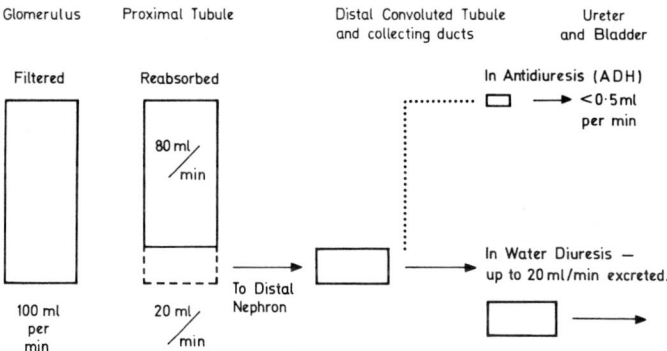

Fig. 9. The fate of the glomerular filtrate. In the proximal tubule, four-fifths of the glomerular filtrate is reabsorbed. About 20 ml per minute reaches the distal tubules and collecting ducts. In a maximal water diuresis, almost all of this volume is excreted. In a maximal antidiuresis, most of it is reabsorbed, and the urine volume is about 0.5 ml per minute.

The ability to produce a small volume of concentrated urine at one point in time and a large volume of dilute urine at another is the result of the following facts:

1. There is an osmotic gradient across the medulla, the outermost regions of which are isotonic with plasma (285

17

m.osm/kg), while the innermost regions are extremely hypertonic (1,200 m.osm/kg at the tips of the renal papilla).

2. In the absence of antidiuretic hormone, the collecting ducts which pass through the medulla are virtually impermeable to water. Sodium is actively reabsorbed from the collecting ducts, but water does not diffuse out to maintain osmotic equilibrium; osmotic forces only act across membranes which are permeable to water. Since sodium is reabsorbed and water is left behind in the tubular lumen, during a water diuresis a large volume of dilute urine is produced.

3. In the presence of antidiuretic hormone the collecting ducts become freely permeable to water. The fluid they contain is exposed to the osmotic forces present in the thirsty medulla. Water is sucked out of the collecting ducts, and the urine which is produced during an antidiuresis is low in volume and high in osmotic concentration.

The concentration gradient which exists across the renal medulla is essential to the production of a hypertonic urine. This concentration gradient is produced and maintained in the following way (Fig. 10).

1. Sodium ions are pumped from the thick segment of the ascending limb of Henle's loop into the medullary interstitium, which becomes slightly hypertonic.

2. A segment of isotonic tubular fluid enters the descending limb of Henle's loop. It equilibrates osmotically with the slightly hypertonic medulla, and becomes slightly hypertonic itself.

3. As this segment of tubular fluid passes down the descending limb, a little sodium is added to it at each point. After a succession of such steps, by the time this fluid has reached the tip of the papilla its osmotic concentration has risen to 1,200 m.osm/kg.

4. This fluid, by now very hypertonic, enters the ascending limb of Henle's loop. At each point in the thick segment sodium is pumped out of it. It becomes progressively more dilute as it passes towards the renal cortex, and is in fact hypotonic by the time it reaches the distal convoluted tubule. The sodium ions it loses are picked up by the fluid in the descending limb and carried down to the tip of the renal papilla, maintaining the osmotic gradient.

5. The vasa recta, like the loops of Henle, form a system of hairpin bends. Fluid in the descending limbs of the vasa recta runs

18

in close proximity to the fluid in the ascending limbs — and in the opposite direction. The blood in the ascending limbs is concentrated. This blood equilibrates with the blood in the descending limbs, picking up water from it, and adding sodium ions to it. This prevents the osmotic gradient across the medulla from being washed out by the medullary circulation.

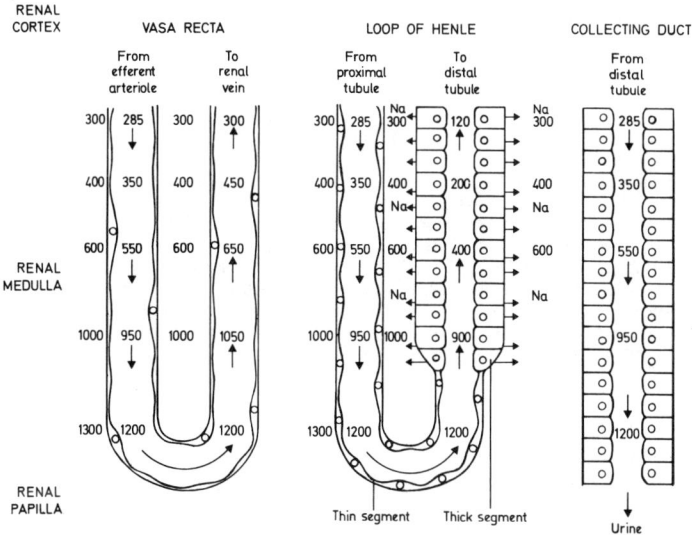

Fig. 10. The countercurrent mechanism in urine concentration. The figures shown on the diagram refer to osmotic concentration in m.osm/kg. Sodium ions are pumped from the lumina of the thick segments of the loops of Henle into the renal interstitium. These ions pass into the descending limbs of the vasa recta and loops of Henle, making the fluid in these limbs more concentrated. Isotonic fluid flowing towards the renal papillae equilibrates osmotically with fluid flowing in the opposite direction. This 'counter-current flow' leads to the formation of an osmotic gradient across the renal medulla.

In the loops of Henle and in the vasa recta the fluid in the descending limbs flows in the opposite direction to that in the ascending limbs. Currents flowing in opposite directions are in close proximity to each other. A system of this kind is known as a counter-current system. The hypothesis outlined above in explaining urinary concentration is a simplified version of what is known as the counter-current hypothesis.

Urea

Between 40 and 70 per cent of urea in the glomerular filtrate is reabsorbed passively by the tubular cells, which are readily permeable to it. Less urea is reabsorbed during a water diuresis because the increased rate of flow allows less time for back diffusion. More urea is reabsorbed during an antidiuresis, not only because there is more time, but also because ADH appears to increase the permeability of cells to urea as well as to water.

FURTHER READING

Berliner. R. W. (1963). Outline of renal physiology. In *Diseases of the Kidney*. Ed. Strauss, M. B. & Welt, L. G. London: Churchill.

Pitts, R. F. (1968). *Physiology of the Kidney and Body Fluids*. 2nd ed. Chicago: Year Book Medical Publishers.

Rhodin, J. (1963). The structure of the kidney. In *Diseases of the Kidney*. Ed. Strauss, M. B. & Welt, L. G. London: Churchill.

Rhodin, J. (1967). Electron microscopy of the kidney. In *Renal Disease*. 2nd ed. Ed. Black, D. A. K. Oxford: Blackwell.

Smith, H. W. (1953). *From Fish to Philosopher*. Boston: Little, Brown.

Chapter 2

ASSESSMENT OF RENAL FUNCTION AND INVESTIGATION OF URINARY TRACT

HISTORY

Some symptoms immediately direct attention to the kidneys or urinary tract. Others, like blurring of vision, nausea, vomiting, muscle weakness, paraesthesia and pleuritic pain (all of which can be caused by disordered renal function) may be confusing unless it is remembered that renal disorders can affect all systems of the body. The taking of a thorough and complete history is as important in diseases of the kidneys and urinary tract as in diseases of any other system.

Pain
Renal pain is felt in the loin (in the angle between the last rib and the sacro-spinalis muscle) or in the hypochondrium. It may be constant, when it is described as 'fixed renal pain', or intermittent, when it is termed renal colic (Fig. 11).

Fixed pain
The renal parenchyma is insensitive, but pain can arise from stretching of the capsule, irritation of the renal pelvis or perinephric inflammation. An enlarged kidney can pull on the nerves of the renal pedicle, while incomplete obstruction of a calyx or the pelvi-ureteric junction can cause pain which is often aggravated by drinking.

Renal and ureteric colic
Colic is, by definition, a pain which occurs in spasms separated by pain-free intervals. Renal colic is a misnomer, because it is a persistent and severe pain with frequent exacerbations. It is caused by sudden and relatively complete obstruction of a calyx, or the pelvi-ureteric junction or of the ureter. The cause of the obstruction is usually a stone or a blood clot.

The pain begins in the loin and radiates to the iliac fossa, the groin, the testis and the penis, or, in women, to the labia. The precise localization depends on the site of the obstruction (Fig. 11). Renal and ureteric colic can be excruciating, and are usually associated with nausea, sweating and restlessness.

Bladder pain

The pain most characteristic of bladder disease is called strangury, and is defined as an urgent and painful desire to pass urine. The pain, which is severe, is felt in the suprapubic region and usually radiates down the urethra to the external meatus. It is caused by spasm of the muscle of the bladder produced by infection of the bladder or prostate, by stones or foreign bodies in the bladder, and by acute retention due to blood clot or any other cause.

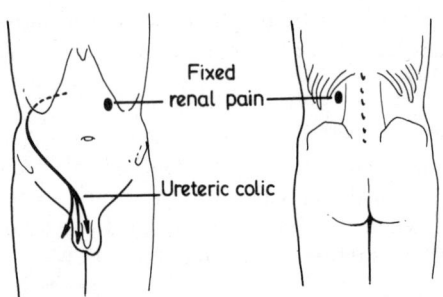

Fig. 11. Fixed renal pain and ureteric colic. Fixed renal pain is located over the kidney, and stays there. Ureteric colic often starts over the kidney, but it radiates from the loin via the flank to the groin.

Prostatic pain

Prostatic pain is felt in the perineum, over the sacrum, in the rectum, or between the thighs. It is usually caused by acute infection of the prostate.

Frequency

The normal bladder capacity is 300 to 400 ml which is the amount of urine passed each time micturition occurs. Voiding usually occurs about once every 3 or 4 hours during the day, and once or not at all during the night.

Increased frequency of micturition may occur:

1. If the total volume of urine produced per 24 hours is excessive; this is called polyuria, and represents an alteration of kidney function.

2. If the amount passed each time is less than the capacity of a normal bladder. This is called 'true frequency' (or simply 'frequency') and is due to altered bladder function.

True frequency may occur from any of the following causes:

1. *Irritation* of the bladder or urethra by infection, stone, foreign body or unaccustomed sexual intercourse.

2. *Contraction* of the bladder by tumour or fibrosis.

3. *Obstruction*. Frequency occurs in obstruction to the outflow tract of the bladder. In the early stages of such obstruction, there may be little residual urine. In the late stages, when there is chronic retention, small quantities of urine overflow from the bladder at frequent intervals.

4. *External pressure.* A pregnant uterus or a large ovarian tumour may compress the bladder and reduce its capacity.

5. *Neurological disease.* Nervous diseases or injuries may interfere with the nerve supply of the bladder and alter its contractility.

6. *Psychological.* The function of the bladder is greatly influenced by the cerebral cortex, and psychological disturbances may cause frequency.

7. *Physiological.* Cold weather and anxiety can cause increased frequency in normal people.

Polyuria

In polyuria the volume of urine passed each time the bladder is emptied is normal, but the total amount of urine passed in 24 hours is greater than normal.

Causes of polyuria

1. Diabetes insipidus. (a) Pituitary (due to lack of secretion of antidiuretic hormone). (b) Nephrogenic (due to inability of kidneys to respond to antidiuretic hormone).

2. Compulsive water drinking.

3. Diabetes mellitus (due to the osmotic effect of excess sugar in the urine).

4. Chronic renal failure (due to the osmotic effect of a large filtered load of urea per functioning nephron, plus loss of renal ability to concentrate the urine).
5. Potassium depletion ⎫ due to impairment of the tubular
6. Hypercalcaemia ⎭ concentrating mechanisms.

Diabetes mellitus can be readily diagnosed by glucose estimations on blood and urine. In *chronic renal failure* the blood urea is raised and the urine contains protein. *Potassium depletion* severe enough to interfere with tubular concentrating mechanisms may also produce proteinuria and a moderate degree of uraemia; estimation of the serum potassium indicates the diagnosis. *Hypercalcaemia* is readily diagnosed by estimation of the serum calcium.

The differentiation of diabetes insipidus from compulsive water drinking is the main diagnostic problem. Water deprivation ultimately causes the compulsive water drinker to produce a reasonably concentrated urine. In diabetes insipidus, on the other hand, water deprivation leads to severe dehydration. The urine remains dilute, but the plasma becomes concentrated. Since patients with diabetes insipidus can become dangerously ill if deprived of water, the test should be carried out only under careful observation, and brought to an end as soon as dehydration becomes apparent.

Nocturia

Rising at night to pass urine may simply be habit and of little clinical importance, but if the patient has not previously had nocturia, or if he passes urine more frequently at night than he used to, the symptom is significant.

Renal handling of salt and water shows a diurnal rhythm, and urine is more concentrated and of smaller volume during the night than in the daytime. If the ability to concentrate the urine is impaired, this diurnal rhythm is abolished. In oedematous patients the normal diurnal rhythm is reversed, because salt and water which accumulate in the dependent parts of the body during the day are reabsorbed into the general circulation at night when the patient is recumbent, and the urine volume increases.

Any patient with frequency or polyuria tends to have nocturia except, perhaps, where the symptoms are of psychological origin. Nocturia is often more noticeable to the patient than frequency occurring during the day.

Haematuria (Fig. 12)

Haematuria is the passage of urine which contains blood. The appearance of such urine varies with the amount of blood and with the hydrogen ion concentration. If the amount of blood is large, the urine is red and thick. It may contain clots. With small

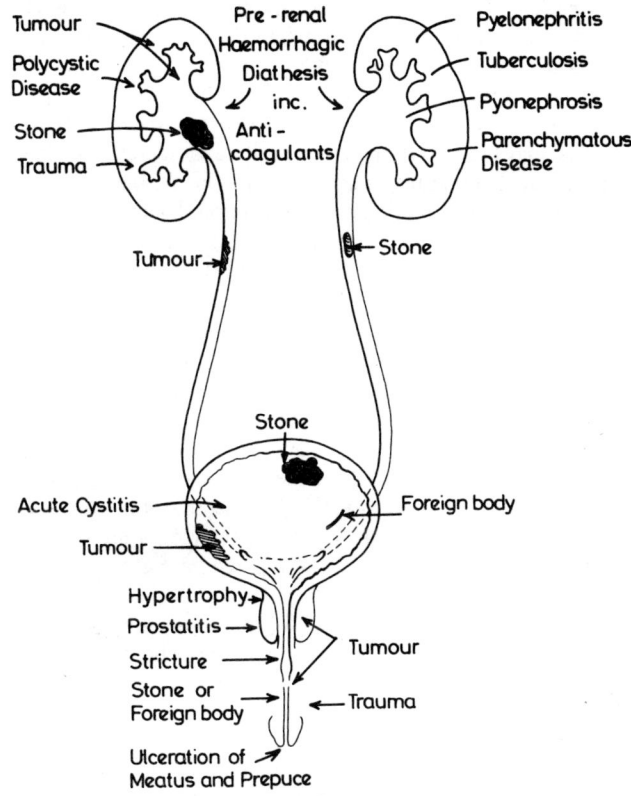

Fig. 12. The causes of haematuria.

to moderate amounts of blood an acid urine appears dark or 'smoky'; in alkaline urine haemoglobin remains red. Since haemoglobin is strongly pigmented, urine which appears normal to the naked eye contains either no blood, or very little.

Chemical stick tests will distinguish colouration due to

25

haemoglobin from that due to substances such as eosin (the colouring agent in many sweets), beetroot, bile or porphyrins. Haematuria can be distinguished from haemoglobinuria by the identification of red blood cells on microscopy.

Haematuria is often intermittent, and a patient who complains of it may have no blood in the urine at the time of examination. Such a patient should generally be investigated on the strength of his history; to ask him to return when the bleeding recurs wastes time – and may on occasion be dangerous.

The blood may be evenly mixed with urine (total haematuria). Alternatively, it may appear either at the beginning of micturition (initial haematuria) or at the end of micturition (terminal haematuria). Total haematuria suggests that the kidney, ureter or bladder is the source, while terminal or initial haematuria suggests the bladder neck, posterior urethra or prostate as its origin. Blood from the distal part of the urethra beyond the sphincter stains the clothes and appears independently of micturition.

The cause of haematuria is often suggested by the symptoms which accompany it. Haematuria occurring with renal colic suggests a stone in the kidney or ureter, but haematuria with elongated blood clots and renal colic suggests a tumour of the kidneys or of the upper urinary tract. Haematuria with frequency and dysuria suggests infection; painless haematuria may indicate a neoplasm of kidney, ureter or bladder. Haematuria which can be detected only on microscopy suggests either some pre-renal cause such as a haemorrhagic diathesis, or a parenchymatous lesion such as glomerulonephritis.

In some patients the cause of haematuria cannot be found, despite careful and repeated investigations. The term 'essential haematuria' is sometimes used to describe such cases.

Haemoglobinuria

Haemoglobin is released by the breakdown of red blood cells within the body. It is bound to large carrier proteins known as haptoglobins, and does not normally appear in the urine. If intravascular haemolysis is marked, however, the haptoglobins become saturated, and free haemoglobin enters the urine. Haemoglobinuria and haematuria are similar in colour and give the same reactions to chemical tests for blood. In haematuria the urine is turbid and red cells can be seen on microscopy. In haemoglobinuria, the urine is not turbid and red cells are absent.

26

EXAMINATION

Physical examination must be systematic and thorough because renal disease can involve every system of the body.

Palpation of the kidneys

One hand is placed on the back below the last rib and lateral to the sacro-spinalis muscle. This hand pushes the kidney forward. The other hand palpates from the front, starting in the iliac fossa and moving upwards. The lower pole of the kidney may be felt during inspiration.

The lower pole of the right kidney, but not of the left, can usually be felt in thin normal subjects who relax well during examination. In obese or anxious patients, however, it may not be possible to feel even abnormally large kidneys.

Kidneys which can be felt easily are either (1) enlarged; (2) displaced by hepatic enlargement, splenic enlargement or retroperitoneal tumours; or (3) excessively mobile. Enlargement of one kidney may be caused by tumour, cyst or hydronephrosis. Alternatively, such enlargement may represent compensatory hypertrophy due to a functionless contralateral kidney. Enlargement of both kidneys is almost always due to polycystic disease.

A palpable right kidney must be distinguished from an enlarged liver, and a palpable left kidney from an enlarged spleen. The kidneys are separated from the anterior abdominal wall by bowel, and percussion over an enlarged kidney will generally reveal areas of resonance. The percussion note over an enlarged liver or spleen is uniformly dull.

Examination of the bladder

In adults the bladder lies in the pelvis and is palpable above the pubic symphysis only if it is distended. A distended bladder produces a midline suprapubic swelling which is dull to percussion. If the retention is acute the swelling is tender and tense, but if the retention is chronic the swelling may be neither tender nor tense and may be surprisingly difficult to detect in an obese patient.

In infants the bladder lies in the abdomen, and even a normal one is often palpable above the pubic symphysis.

The external genitalia

Penis. The prepuce often obscures lesions of the glans, and

27

must always be retracted, unless it is phimotic, and replaced after the glans has been examined. (Phimosis is excessive tightness of the foreskin.) Phimosis or a meatal stricture may obstruct the outflow of urine from the bladder and lead to distension of the bladder, hydronephrosis and other consequences of obstruction.

Scrotal contents. A systematic examination must be made of the testes, the epididymes, the spermatic cords and their coverings. A tuberculous epididymitis may confirm a suspicion of renal tuberculosis. A left varicocele may suggest a renal carcinoma invading the renal vein on that side. A testicular tumour may explain enlargement of neck or paravertebral lymph nodes, while a congenital anomaly of testis or penis may suggest that another congenital anomaly is the cause of renal, ureteric or bladder symptoms.

Female genitalia. The female genitalia can be assessed adequately only by vaginal examination. This is most easily carried out under anaesthesia and in urological practice is often done immediately after cystoscopy.

EXAMINATION OF THE URINE

Chemical testing of the urine has been greatly simplified by the introduction of impregnated paper strips which detect substances such as glucose, acetone, bilirubin, protein and blood.

Of particular importance in renal disease are:
1. The detection of protein in the urine.
2. The measurement of the urine specific gravity or osmolality.
3. The microscopic examination of the urine for red blood cells, white blood cells and casts.

Examination of the urine for protein

The most widely used test for proteinuria is the 'stick test'. A strip of paper impregnated with a buffer and the indicator bromophenol blue turns green if dipped into urine that contains protein. The test depends on the principle that protein interferes with the normal relationship between pH and the colour of the indicator. Because it may give misleading results in strongly alkaline or strongly acid urine, and because it does not always detect Bence-Jones protein (found in some patients with myeloma), the

28

salicyl-sulphonic acid test is often preferred. A 25 per cent solution of salicyl-sulphonic acid produces turbidity when added to urine that contains 20 mg per cent of any protein, and a flocculant precipitate if there is heavy proteinuria. If the urine contains protein, the total excretion in 24 hours should be measured, using an aliquot from a 24-hour collection, the volume of which is known. The Esbach method consists of measuring the amount of protein precipitated by a picric acid/citric acid mixture, using a tube specially calibrated to record the protein concentration directly from the amount of precipitate. It is not a very accurate test. More satisfactory is the biuret reaction, which is a colorimetric test that can be carried out only in a clinical chemistry laboratory.

Estimation of the specific gravity of urine

The specific gravity of urine is measured with a hydrometer. If urine passed first thing in the morning before the patient has drunk anything has a specific gravity of 1025 or more, the concentrating power of kidneys can be regarded as normal, provided that the urine contains neither sugar nor protein.

Urine microscopy

This is most conveniently carried out on a centrifuged specimen, the deposit from which is resuspended in 0.5 ml of urine. Centrifugation should be carried out at the slowest practicable speed since casts are disrupted by rapid centrifugation. Urine from a normal subject treated in this way will contain at most 1 or 2 red blood cells and 3 or 4 white blood cells per high power field. Several fields will have to be scanned before a cast is seen.

Quantitative counts of the cells and casts in urine by the Addis technique can be performed, but the procedure is time-consuming and inaccurate except when done by an expert.

Red blood cells appear under the microscope as pale, yellowish rings − crenated if the urine is concentrated, and swollen if the urine is dilute. In very dilute urine red cells rupture and only the shreds of cell membranes can be seen.

White blood cells are larger than red cells and have a central granular appearance.

Large flat cells are often seen in urine specimens from female patients. These are derived from the vagina.

Casts are formed in the renal tubules by the agglutination of albumin with a tubular muco-protein, Tamm Horsfall protein. They take on the shape of the tubules where they form. *Hyaline casts* are structureless and large numbers may be seen in the urine of patients with proteinuria. *Red cell casts* are formed by the incorporation of erythrocytes derived from the glomeruli into hyaline casts. They are seen in glomerulonephritis and occasionally in malignant hypertension. *Granular casts* occur in many renal diseases, including glomerulonephritis. They are formed by the incorporation of red blood cells and desquamated, degenerate tubular cells into hyaline casts.

Urine contains a great many crystals. Only amino-acid crystals are of clinical importance, and amino-aciduria is more readily diagnosed by chemical means than by microscopy.

THE ASSESSMENT OF GLOMERULAR FUNCTION

Blood urea. The normal range for blood urea is 15 to 35 mg per 100 ml. As the glomerular filtration rate falls, the blood urea level rises, but the rise is barely detectable until filtration has fallen to 30–40 per cent of normal. The rate of urea production is as important as the rate of elimination in determining the blood urea level. Excessive protein breakdown can arise from a high protein diet, or from excessive catabolism of body proteins. Infection, steroid therapy and blood in the gastro-intestinal tract raise the blood urea level, while a high fluid intake reduces it. The blood urea is therefore only an approximate index of glomerular function.

Creatinine clearance. In the dog, creatinine is neither secreted nor reabsorbed by the renal tubules, and determination of the creatinine clearance gives a true measure of the glomerular filtration rate. In man, a small amount of creatinine is secreted by the renal tubules, but in spite of this, creatinine clearance determinations give a measure of glomerular filtration which is adequate for most clinical purposes. Measurement of the creatinine clearance involves the accurate collection of a 24-hour urine specimen, and the taking of a blood specimen, ideally at the mid-point of the collection period.

If for research purposes it is necessary to measure the

glomerular filtration rate more precisely, inulin clearances are determined.

ASSESSMENT OF TUBULAR FUNCTION

1. Tests of tubular concentrating ability

The concentration of urine can be assessed by measuring either its specific gravity or osmotic pressure. The specific gravity is proportional to the solute concentration in g/100 ml, whereas osmotic pressure, which depends on the number of particles in solution, is proportional to the solute concentration in mEq/litre. Protein and glucose are large molecules and contribute much to specific gravity but little to osmotic pressure. Nevertheless, if a morning specimen of urine has a specific gravity of 1.025 and contains neither protein nor glucose, there can be little wrong with the concentrating ability of the kidneys.

A more accurate test involves the use of vasopressin combined with water deprivation. The bladder is emptied 14 hours after the patient has been deprived of food and drink, and 8 hours after an injection of 10 units of vasopressin, and the urine is discarded. Hourly specimens of urine are then obtained for 2 hours. The osmolality of 1 of the 2 specimens should be 800 m.osm/kg or more.

2. Tests of tubular diluting ability

The tubular diluting ability can be assessed by a water load test. A fasting patient is given 20 ml of water for each kilogram of his body weight in 20 minutes, and urine is collected at hourly intervals for 4 hours. The specific gravity should be 1.004 or less in at least 1 of the hourly specimens, and at least 75 per cent of the water load should be excreted in 4 hours. If the patient is agitated or nauseated, however, anti-diuretic hormone may be secreted and invalidate the result. The test may cause water intoxication in patients who are unable to excrete a water load and who may already have dilute body fluids before the test starts. The ability to dilute urine is lost early in Addison's disease, but late in most renal diseases:

3. Tests of renal ability to control acid base balance

The ability of the kidney to excrete hydrogen ions (H^+) can be assessed by loading the body with acid. If the patient is already acidotic it is unnecessary to give more acid. The pH of a fresh specimen of urine is measured; unless this is 5.3 or less, the kidneys' ability to excrete H^+ is impaired.

If the patient is not acidotic, an acid load is administered as ammonium chloride (0.1 g/kg body weight). Ammonium chloride is metabolized to urea with the production of hydrochloric acid:

$$2 NH_4Cl + CO_2 = CO (NH_2)_2 + H_2O + 2 HCl$$

Hourly specimens of urine are taken for 7 hours and collected into containers containing a small amount of liquid paraffin, which preserves bicarbonate. In at least 1 of the 7 specimens the pH should be less than 5.3; the titratable acidity should be more than 25 μEq/min and the excretion of ammonia more than 35 μEq/min.

4. Tubular ability to conserve sodium

Normal kidneys can produce urine that contains no more than 0.5 mEq/l of sodium. In renal disease the ability to conserve sodium may be lost and some patients suffer sodium depletion. Sodium depletion can be readily recognized by the effects it has on the circulation and by the improvement in these effects and on the glomerular filtration rate that follows the administration of sodium salts. The confirmation of tubular inability to conserve sodium may on occasion involve sodium balance studies. On a low sodium diet (10 mEq per day) sodium excretion normally falls to equal sodium intake within a week. Failure to retain sodium may be due to Addison's disease and not to renal tubular impairment, and Addison's disease should be excluded before salt deprivation is carried out.

5. Tubular ability to conserve potassium

Potassium depletion due to renal disease is seen in association with inability to acidify the urine in renal tubular acidosis and in the Fanconi syndrome. Increased aldosterone production, whether due to primary adrenal disease or secondary to conditions such as cardiac failure or ascites, can also lead to potassium depletion. The clinical context will usually explain a low serum potassium level, but on occasion it is necessary to embark on protracted potassium balance studies involving unappetizing low potassium diets.

RADIOLOGY OF THE KIDNEYS AND
URINARY TRACT

Modern radiographic techniques give not only detailed information of the structure of the kidneys and urinary tract, but also useful, if approximate, information regarding function.

Straight X-rays of renal tract

A straight X-ray of the renal tract must include the diaphragm above and the pubic symphysis below, even if two films are required.

The renal outlines are usually visible and can be measured. The ureters cannot be seen, nor the bladder unless it is distended, when it appears as a soft tissue shadow in the pelvis. The lateral borders of the psoas major muscles are normally visible. If one is obscured this suggests a perinephric abscess, a psoas abscess or an enlarged kidney. Calcification in the kidneys, bladder or prostate is visible, as are stones (other than uric acid and cystine ones), unless they lie over bone or are very small. Opacities in the renal tract must be distinguished from gall-stones, calcified costal cartilages, phleboliths (calcified thrombi in the pelvic veins) and calcified fibroids. All structures shown in the films must be looked at; the finding of osteomalacia or of metastases in the bones may tell more than could ever be learned by looking at the structures of the urinary tract.

Intravenous pyelography

An intravenous pyelogram is probably the most useful investigation of the urinary tract. Organic iodine compounds are radio-opaque. When given by intravenous injection they are excreted by the kidneys. If they are concentrated sufficiently in the process of excretion, they can be seen radiologically. Excretion is predominantly by glomerular filtration with little tubular secretion. It reaches a maximum some 8 to 12 minutes after injection, then gradually diminishes until nearly all the iodine has been excreted, usually 60 to 90 minutes after injection. The *amount* excreted and the speed with which it passes through the tubules depend upon glomerular filtration rate, but the *concentration,* which determines the density of the dye and therefore the opacity of the kidney and urinary tract, varies inversely with the volume of water excreted. The patient is deprived of fluid for

6 hours before the test, and instructed to take a laxative 2 days before the test so that the kidneys will not be obscured by gas or faeces in the bowel. The dye may pass through the calyces and pelvis so quickly that their outline cannot be clearly demonstrated. Better filling of pelves and calcyes is obtained if the ureters are partly obstructed during the early films by inflating a pneumatic belt strapped to the abdomen. The ureters and bladder can be studied in films made after the compression is released, usually 25, 30 or 40 minutes after injection. If another film is taken after the patient has passed urine, the amount of residual urine, if any, that remains in the bladder after micturition can be assessed. If there is obstruction late films (6, 12, 24, or even 48 hours after injection) should be taken, because obstruction reduces not only the rate of glomerular filtration but also the rate at which the filtrate passes through the tubules and urinary tract. Sufficient dye to produce a picture may reach pelvis or calyces or ureter only after many hours.

The dye used is sodium diatrizoate, and it appears to have no deleterious action on the kidney even when active disease is present. Some patients, usually with known allergies, are hypersensitive to it, but even they can have intravenous pyelograms provided that the injection is given slowly and hydrocortisone or antihistamines are available for immediate use if a reaction occurs.

Chronic renal failure may be a contra-indication to intravenous pyelography, not because the dye will damage the kidneys, but because the kidneys will not concentrate the dye sufficiently to produce pictures. In these cases satisfactory pictures may be obtained if two or three times the normal dose is given either by injection or by infusion over half-an-hour.

Retrograde pyelography

Retrograde pyelograms are X-rays made after the injection of an iodine-containing compound into the pelvis of the kidney through a catheter previously passed up the ureters at cystoscopy. If a ureterogram is required the dye can be injected through a catheter with a solid bulb some 0.5 cm below its tip. The bulb prevents the injected dye from leaking back into the bladder before the examination has been concluded.

Retrograde pyelography is uncomfortable and may introduce or spread infection. It is justifiable only if an intravenous pyelogram does not show sufficient detail of the pelvis, calyces and ureter.

Aortography

The renal blood vessels can be visualized by the injection of contrast media into the aorta, or (if one is more interested in one kidney than the other) by injection of contrast medium into the renal artery concerned. It is usually carried out by retrograde percutaneous femoral catheterization. The main value of aortography is the determination of structural anomalies, such as stenosis of the main renal vessels, and abnormal vascular circulations in the kidney, like those found in tumours.

Cystography

If an intravenous pyelogram does not show the bladder in sufficient detail, a cystogram can be carried out in the following manner:

300 ml of 12.5 per cent sterile sodium iodide solution is injected into the bladder through a catheter. Organic iodine compounds can be used but are expensive and unnecessary because little if any dye is absorbed from the bladder. X-rays are taken in the antero-posterior plane and in such other planes as seem necessary. Tumours appear as filling defects; diverticula as pouches filled with dye. If further X-rays are taken during micturition, dye outlines the bladder neck and urethra and may reflux into the ureters. A cystogram is usually essential for the investigation of diverticula and the detection of vesico-ureteric reflux.

Urethrography

X-ray pictures of the urethra can be taken during a voiding cystogram. More detailed films can be obtained after injection of an organic iodine solution or gel directly into the urethra through a syringe, the tip of which is inserted into the external meatus.

Presacral air insufflation

Oxygen or carbon dioxide can be injected into the retroperitoneal tissues through a needle inserted under local anaesthesia, between the sacrum and the anal canal. When the patient sits or stands up the gas ascends and surrounds the kidneys and adrenals, which can then be easily identified in X-rays. This method of examination is of more value in adrenal than in renal disease.

Endoscopic procedures
Cystoscopy

A cystoscope is an instrument that can be passed through the urethra into the bladder under local or general anaesthesia. It allows the interior of the bladder to be viewed with the same facility as one can inspect skin with the naked eye.

The cystoscope is passed and the bladder emptied. 300 ml of sterile water or saline is introduced and the bladder examined. If there is much bleeding during the bladder examination, the saline opacifies and vision is difficult. A biopsy of any suspicious lesion can be taken using Lowsley forceps or a resectoscope. The ureters can be catheterized and retrograde pyelograms made. Urine can be collected separately from each kidney for differential renal function tests and for bacteriological examination.

Urethroscopy

Although the prostatic urethra can often be examined through an ordinary cystoscope, to examine the rest of the urethra a slightly different instrument called a urethroscope is needed.

BIOPSY

Percutaneous renal biopsy

Percutaneous renal biopsy is the most convenient way of carrying out a specific morphological evaluation of diffuse renal disease during life. The main indication for renal biopsy is for the diagnosis of diffuse renal disease where clinical, biochemical or X-ray procedures have proved inconclusive. The procedure is dangerous in patients who are unco-operative, who have coagulation disorders or who have a solitary kidney. In patients with perinephric abscesses or renal tumours renal biopsy is absolutely contraindicated. The specimens obtained should be examined by both light and electron microscopy.

Bladder biopsy

This can readily be carried out during cystoscopy, using Lowsley forceps or a resectoscope.

Prostatic biopsy

Prostatic biopsy is sometimes carried out in patients with

possible malignant disease of the prostate, where the diagnosis cannot be confirmed by clinical, biochemical or X-ray procedures. The biopsy can be taken either by open operation through the perineum or retro-pubic space, or through the anterior wall of the rectum, using a Vim-Silverman needle or a pituitary rongeur.

Testicular biopsy

A biopsy can be taken from the testis through a small incision in the tunica albuginea. This method of biopsy is used only in the investigation of infertility. Suspected testicular tumours should never be biopsied, they should be excised.

Isotope renography

Hippuric acid derivatives are filtered at the glomeruli and secreted by the tubules. Hippuran can be labelled with ^{131}I, a radioactive iodine isotope. If this labelled material is injected intravenously, a geiger-counter placed over the kidneys will record the appearance and disappearance of radioactivity in the kidneys. The rate at which the isotope appears in the kidney gives an indication of renal blood flow. Delayed disappearance of radioactivity from the kidney is indicative of obstruction (Fig. 13).

Isotope scanning of the kidney

A radioactive isotope of mercury which is actively taken up by renal tubular cells is given intravenously. A moving sensor traverses the abdomen, and a 'map' is drawn electronically, relating the intensity of radiation to certain surface landmarks. Provided renal function is adequate, the shape of the kidneys can readily be made out. Tumours and cysts show up as 'cold' areas, devoid of radioactivity.

BACTERIOLOGICAL EXAMINATIONS

Catheter specimens of urine

If the bladder has to be catheterized to relieve obstruction, or for some similar reason, catheter specimens of urine should be sent for culture. To catheterize the bladder solely to obtain an uncontaminated specimen of urine, however, is rarely justifiable, as the procedure can introduce infection, or lead to the spread of infection which is already present.

Midstream specimens of urine

Satisfactory 'clean-catch' specimens of urine can be obtained from any reasonably co-operative patient. After cleaning the penis or vulva, the patient is instructed to micturate — holding the labia apart, in the case of female patients. A few seconds after the start of micturition, a sterile container is introduced into the

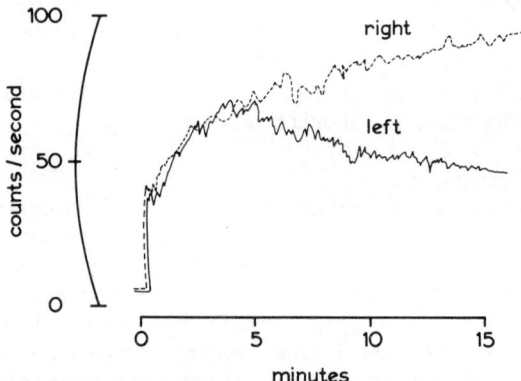

Fig. 13. An [131]I Hippuran renogram, showing a normal left kidney and an obstructed right kidney. The rising part of the curve represents the arrival of the isotope at the kidney in the renal artery, and its accumulation within the kidney during glomerular filtration and tubular secretion. The falling part of the curve is the excretory phase, showing removal of the isotope from the kidney in the urine. In the obstructed right kidney, the isotope is not excreted normally, and the tracing continues to rise, showing continued accumulation of the isotope.

urinary stream. The first part of the urine stream washes out the organisms from the urethra and adjacent genitalia; the midstream specimen is therefore *relatively* free of contamination. It is not absolutely free of extraneous organisms and in practice organisms present in amounts of 10^5 per ml or less are disregarded as contaminants, while counts of 10^6 or over are held to indicate active infection of the bladder, the kidneys or both. Counts of between 10^5 and 10^6 per ml are equivocal, and are an indication for a repeat examination.

Interpretation of the bacterial count is helped by microscopy of the centrifuged deposit from the specimen. The presence of abundant pus cells is in favour of active infection, while the presence of vaginal squames in any number suggests contamination of the specimen from the genital tract. The finding of pus cells in sterile urine suggests tuberculosis.

Supra-pubic puncture of the bladder

It is not at all easy to obtain an uncontaminated midstream specimen of urine from infants. In infants, however, the bladder lies in the abdomen. A needle can be inserted into it through the lower part of the abdominal wall, and urine can be aspirated directly from the bladder. This is an easy procedure, and carries much less risk of introducing infection than bladder catheterization.

Needle aspiration of bladder urine is rather more difficult in adults, since the bladder is a pelvic organ. Provided the bladder is full, however, the technique is feasible, but since most adults can provide satisfactory midstream specimens, it is seldom necessary.

Blood culture

Any patient with a severe urinary tract infection associated with high fever or with rigors should have blood taken for culture. Bacteraemia occurs fairly often in this context. Occasionally, when infection occurs in an obstructed kidney, the urine is sterile, and blood culture may be the most rapid way of reaching a bacteriological diagnosis.

Diagnosis of urinary tuberculosis

If tuberculosis is suspected (as in unexplained haematuria or sterile pyuria), urine should be cultured for the tubercle bacillus. Tubercle bacilli do not appear in large numbers in the urine, even when the disease is active, and culture of an ordinary midstream specimen will, as a rule fail to reveal the organism. A relatively large amount of urine must be sent to the laboratory if tuberculosis is suspected. It is usual to take the whole of the first urine specimen passed in the morning for this purpose.

Syphilis is a relatively rare cause of renal tract disease; if it is suspected, blood should be taken for the Wassermann reaction.

Gonorrhoea is a much more common venereal disease. It is best diagnosed by the demonstration of Gram-negative intracellular diplococci in a specimen of urethral discharge. The gonococcus is a delicate organism, and successful culture depends on the rapid transfer of the specimen to the laboratory in a suitable transport medium.

Blainey, J. D. (1965). Estimation of the glomerular filtration rate. *J. clin. Path.*, **18**, 511.

Muehrcke, R. & Pirani, C. L. (1967). Percutaneous renal biopsy. In *Renal Disease*, 2nd ed. Ed. Black, D. A. K. Oxford: Blackwell.

Relman, A. S. & Levinsky, N. G. (1963). Clinical examination of renal function. In *Diseases of the Kidney*. Ed. Strauss, M. B. & Welt, L. G. London: Churchill.

Wrong, O. & Davies, H. E. F. (1959). The excretion of acid in renal disease. *Q. Jl Med.*, N.S. **28**, 259.

Chapter 3

DISORDERS OF THE RENAL PARENCHYMA

GLOMERULONEPHRITIS

Glomerulonephritis is disease which primarily affects the glomeruli.

Classification

Early attempts to classify glomerulonephritis were both numerous and confusing. Ellis improved the situation considerably when he introduced a classification based on the careful clinical observation of several hundred cases.

In *Ellis Type I nephritis* the onset is acute and often preceded by a sore throat. The features are haematuria, proteinuria, oedema, hypertension and oliguria: 90 per cent of cases recover.

In *Ellis Type II nephritis* the onset is insidious and a history of a preceding acute attack is rarely obtained. The main feature of the disease is proteinuria, usually associated with oedema. Recovery is unusual, and patients tend to progress to chronic renal failure.

The Ellis classification is a *clinical* one. Renal biopsy allows the examination of renal tissue by both light and electron microscopy at an early stage in the disease process, and has made it possible to define 3 fairly clear-cut *pathological* entities, *proliferative glomerulonephritis, membranous glomerulonephritis* and *minimal lesion glomerulonephritis.*

All patients with an Ellis Type I nephritis have proliferative changes on histological examination.

Patients with Ellis Type II nephritis may have minimal, membranous or proliferative glomerulonephritis or conditions like renal amyloidosis or renal vein thrombosis.

Histological Appearances

1. Proliferative glomerulonephritis

In proliferative glomerulonephritis the pathological process affects predominantly the endothelial cells of the glomerulus which swell and increase in number. Fibrin adheres to the glomerular capillary wall and damages the basement membrane, which becomes irregularly thickened. Protein and red and white blood cells escape through the damaged basement membrane into the tubular space of Bowman's capsule and form deposits which are called crescents because of their shape. If the disease progresses the glomeruli are obliterated by endothelial cell proliferation, crescent formation and fibrin deposition. The glomeruli and tubules are deprived of their blood supply, and replaced by fibrous tissue.

2. Membranous glomerulonephritis

In membranous glomerulonephritis there is marked thickening of the capillary basement membrane, with little cellular proliferation. The thickened basement membrane narrows and eventually obliterates the lumina of the glomerular capillaries. The glomeruli and tubules, deprived of their blood supply, are replaced by fibrous tissue.

3. Minimal lesion glomerulonephritis

In minimal lesion glomerulonephritis the kidney appears normal on light microscopy. On electron microscopy, however, the changes are characteristic. The foot processes of the epithelial cells of Bowman's capsule (Fig. 14) disintegrate, and remain only as a thin smear of protoplasm applied to the capsular side of the basement membrane. Similar changes in foot processes are sometimes seen in both proliferative and membranous glomerulonephritis and appear to be the result of proteinuria, but only in minimal lesion glomerulonephritis are these changes uniform and extensive.

Acute Glomerulonephritis

Acute glomerulonephritis corresponds to Ellis Type I nephritis.

Aetiology

This condition is often preceded by streptococcal infection, usually of the tonsils, but sometimes of the skin, the middle ear or other sites. The streptococcus is Lancefield Group A, and

42

often Griffiths type 4 or 12. The organism itself cannot be recovered from the renal lesions, and probably causes nephritis by an immune mechanism.

An experimental type of renal disease called Masugi nephritis can be produced in normal rats by the injection of serum taken from rabbits immunized against rat glomeruli. It closely resembles

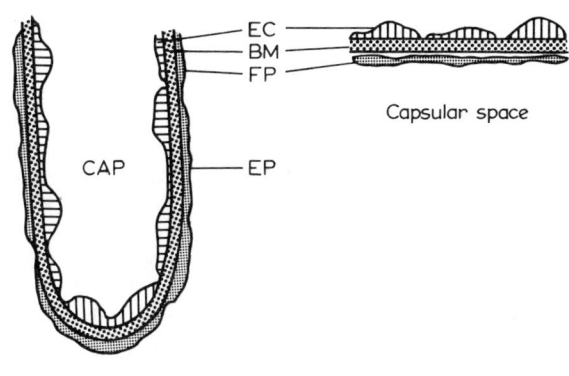

Capsular space

Fig. 14. Electron microscope appearances in minimal lesion glomerulonephritis. The basement membrane appears entirely normal, but there has been loss of the structure of the epithelial foot processes which are represented by a continuous layer of protoplasm applied to the epithelial surface of the basement membrane. (Cf Fig. 2.)

acute nephritis in man, both clinically and pathologically. It is possible that antigens produced by the streptococcus are similar to antigens present in the glomerular basement membrane, and that antibodies produced against streptococci react not only with the infecting organisms but also with the host's own glomeruli. An alternative explanation is that host antibody and bacterial antigen react to produce an insoluble antigen-antibody complex which is deposited on the basement membrane, and which produces an inflammatory reaction in the glomeruli.

Pathology

The pathology is that of proliferative glomerulonephritis. The changes are usually diffuse, but are sometimes focal. In moderately severe cases there may be necrosis of a few glomeruli with a variable amount of tubular degeneration and interstitial inflammation. In severe cases there is often widespread fibrin deposition in the glomeruli, marked crescent formation and diffuse interstitial inflammation. The severity of the changes in the glomeruli correlates with the severity of the clinical symptoms and gives a good index of ultimate prognosis.

Lesions similar to those seen in acute glomerulonephritis of streptococcal origin are also seen in anaphylactoid purpura, polyarteritis, systemic lupus erythematosus and Goodpasture's syndrome. These conditions can have a similar clinical presentation and are probably also caused by immunological mechanisms.

Clinical features

Acute glomerulonephritis is predominantly a disease of children and young adults. The onset is abrupt, and in typical cases occurs some 10 to 14 days after a streptococcal throat or skin infection. It is characterized by haematuria, proteinuria, hypertension, oedema and oliguria. Many of these features may be absent, and mild cases may simply have proteinuria, a slight reduction in urine volume and slight haematuria.

Proteinuria is a constant feature of glomerular damage. In acute nephritis its degree is variable. It may be simply an observation on urine testing, or be of sufficient magnitude to deplete the plasma proteins and produce the nephrotic syndrome.

Haematuria may be readily visible, or may be detected only on microscopic examination of the urine. It may be the only obvious feature of the disease, especially in young children.

Oliguria. Swelling and proliferation of the glomerular endothelial cells reduce glomerular filtration. The tubules are normal (at least in the early stages) and reabsorb a large proportion of the reduced amount of filtrate. The urine tends to be concentrated, and of low volume.

Oedema is due to salt and water retention and a slight generalized increase in capillary permeability. If massive proteinuria persists for a number of weeks, hypoproteinaemia will occur, and this will also contribute to the oedema.

Hypertension is usually moderate, and more prominent in adults than in children. A sudden rise in blood pressure, or sustained hypertension, may lead to hypertensive encephalopathy or to acute left ventricular failure.

Renal failure. In severe cases renal function may be markedly impaired. Glomerular function is affected more than tubular

44

function. The creatinine clearance is reduced and the blood urea level elevated. In some patients the urine output declines to complete anuria over a period of a week to 10 days, and in fulminant cases anuria may occur at the onset of the illness. Not all patients with renal failure have irreversible renal damage. Cases have been recorded in which complete recovery followed a period of anuria lasting for more than 6 weeks.

Investigations

The streptococcal aetiology should be confirmed if possible, since other conditions may produce a similar clinical picture. A history of sore throat, scarlet fever or other streptococcal manifestation should be sought. Throat swabs should be taken, and Lancefield grouping carried out on any streptococci found. The antistreptolysin O titre in serum is a useful investigation. It is normally between 100 and 200 Todd units, but in patients with recent streptococcal infections it is often 800 or more Todd units per ml. X-rays of teeth and sinuses should be taken, as these sites may harbour hidden foci of infection.

Treatment

Penicillin. If streptococci persist in the body they tend to keep the immunological process going. It is therefore reasonable to treat acute nephritis with penicillin.

Bed rest is a vital part of therapy and ideally should continue until red cells and protein have disappeared from the urine. In practice, patients are often allowed up after about 3 weeks provided they feel well, because proteinuria and haematuria can persist for many months even in patients who eventually make a complete recovery.

Salt and water restriction. Water intoxication, cardiac failure and other complications such as hypertension can be largely prevented by limiting the intake of salt and water. In all but the mildest cases, the fluid intake should be limited to 500 ml plus the volume of the previous day's output, and the sodium intake limited to 0.5 g to 1.0 g daily.

Acute left ventricular failure is nearly always secondary to overhydration and can generally be prevented by restricting salt and water intake. If it occurs, digoxin, morphine and (if the kidneys can respond) diuretics should be used. Salt and water can also be removed from the body by dialysis (Chap. 5). Venesection is sometimes life-saving.

'Hypertensive encephalopathy' may occur because the high blood pressure causes spasm of the cerebral vessels. The neurological features vary. Status epilepticus is relatively common and potentially dangerous. During an epileptic convulsion, there is transient respiratory obstruction, which causes respiratory acidosis. Hydrogen ions accumulate in the body and displace potassium from the cells into the plasma. A high serum potassium level can cause cardiac arrest, particularly if renal function is impaired. Convulsions complicating renal disease should always be brought under control urgently with anticonvulsants such as phenobarbitone and Epanutin, and the blood pressure should be restored to normal levels with parenteral, fast-acting drugs (Chap. 6).

Renal failure. If renal failure supervenes, treatment is as described in Chapter 4.

Prognosis

Ninety per cent of patients with acute glomerulonephritis make a complete recovery. Of the remaining 10 per cent, about a quarter either die of hypertension or cardiac failure early in the disease, or progress rapidly to irreversible renal failure, while the rest have persistent proteinuria and persistent hypertension, and progress to renal failure over a period of months or years.

THE NEPHROTIC SYNDROME

Introduction

The nephrotic syndrome is characterized by proteinuria, oedema, a low plasma protein concentration and an increased blood cholesterol content. It corresponds roughly to what Ellis termed Type II nephritis, and occurs at some stage in many renal diseases.

Glomerular damage renders the basement membrane abnormally permeable to protein, and the loss of protein in the urine lowers the plasma protein concentration. The plasma protein osmotic pressure is one of the factors responsible for keeping fluid in the vascular compartment, and the low serum protein concentration allows salt and water to leave the circulation and accumulate in the interstitial space. The lowered blood volume

46

activates volume receptors in the larger blood vessels. This leads, among other things, to an increased production of aldosterone, and the retention of salt and water. The blood volume is not restored to normal, however, because much of the extra salt and water that is retained in the body escapes into the interstitial spaces, and increases the oedema.

Oedema can be quite massive; one nephrotic patient weighed 110 kg before treatment, but only 50 kg after the excess fluid was eliminated.

Aetiology

Any renal disorder that is associated with marked proteinuria can produce the nephrotic syndrome. Of 705 patients with the nephrotic syndrome reviewed by Robson, 77 per cent had primary glomerulonephritis (membranous in 30 per cent, proliferative in 22 per cent, minimal lesion in 18 per cent and mixed membranous and proliferative in 7 per cent). In the other 23 per cent the renal damage was caused by diseases such as systemic lupus erythematosus (SLE), renal amyloidosis, diabetic nephropathy and renal vein thrombosis. Exponents of listmanship can produce about 75 causes for the nephrotic syndrome, but the ones mentioned above are the most important and account for over 90 per cent of cases in this country. Malaria due to *Plasmodium malariae* is an important cause of the nephrotic syndrome in areas where malaria due to this organism is endemic. Symptomless proteinuria may either be caused by the same diseases that cause the nephrotic syndrome, or be postural. Postural proteinuria is a benign condition and is described on page 63.

Proteinuria

This is an almost invariable feature of diseases of the renal parenchyma. Bright and Bostock were the first to describe the relationship between renal disease and proteinuria in detail, but the relationship between proteinuria and oedema was noted by Cottunius in the 18th century.

Some protein is filtered through normal glomeruli and re-absorbed in the proximal convoluted tubule. The amount filtered in man is not known, but animal experiments suggest that it is about 20 mg per 100 ml, which is very much less than the concentration of protein in the plasma (7.0 g per 100 ml). Tubular secretion of protein does not occur, but trace amounts of protein are added to urine in the tubules and urinary tract from the breakdown of epithelial cells.

Small proteins, such as haemoglobin and some of the abnormal proteins produced in multiple myeloma, pass through normal glomeruli. In the nephrotic syndrome, however, protein-uria is always caused by increased glomerular permeability to protein. The glomerulus can be regarded as a filter with 'holes' small enough to prevent all but a tiny proportion of plasma protein from passing through into the capsular space. If the basement membrane is damaged, these 'holes' enlarge and protein passes through more easily. If the amount of protein filtered exceeds the tubular reabsorptive capacity, protein appears in the urine.

'Selectivity' of the glomerular filter

In minimal lesion glomerulonephritis, the holes are only slightly larger than normal and the glomerulus behaves as a selective filter, holding back all but the smallest protein molecules. The filtration of large protein molecules is still impeded, and the clearance of albumin (molecular weight 69,000) is about 1,000 times the clearance of alpha 2 globulin (molecular weight 800,000).

In membranous glomerulonephritis, the damage to the glomerulus is more severe and the holes are larger. The glomerulus behaves as an unselective filter. Large proteins pass through (though less readily than small ones) and the albumin clearance is only 10 to 100 times the alpha 2 globulin clearance. Differential protein clearance determinations show whether the glomerulus is behaving as a selective or an unselective filter, provided that the protein has passed through the glomerulus and has not been added to the urine in the renal pelvis or bladder in the form of pus or blood. If the protein excretion pattern is selective, the glomerular damage is likely to be slight, and there is a good chance of a favourable response to steroid therapy. Patients with unselective proteinuria hardly ever respond well to steroid therapy.

Clinical features of the nephrotic syndrome

The patient may be of any age or either sex. The principal clinical feature is oedema, which tends to come on gradually and to fluctuate in severity. The cause of the oedema is the loss of

48

protein in the urine, but the amount of protein lost does not correlate precisely with the severity of the oedema, because people vary in their ability to make good the protein lost by protein synthesis. Oedema gravitates to the dependent parts. It is most marked in the feet and ankles during the day, and in the soft tissues around the eyes in the morning when the patient awakes. In severe cases, fluid accumulates in many sites and ascites and pleural effusions occur.

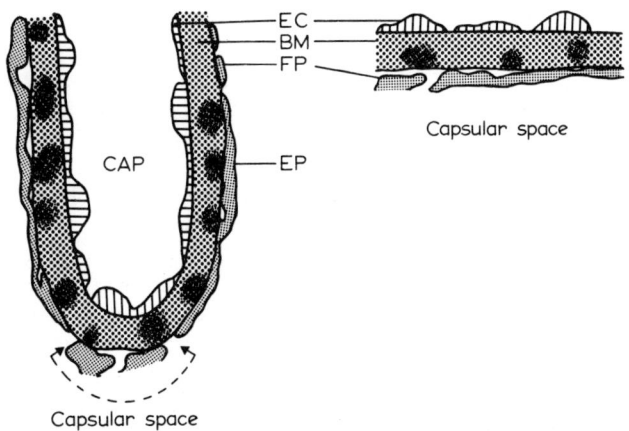

Fig. 15. Electron microscope appearances in membranous glomerulonephritis. The basement membrane is thickened, and there are deposits of electron dense material on its epithelial aspect. There is in addition some loss of structure of the epithelial foot processes. (Cf. Fig. 2.)

Patients with the nephrotic syndrome are very susceptible to infection, and in pre-antibiotic days often died from cellulitis, peritonitis, pneumonia or empyema.

The patient's clinical course depends on the cause of the nephrotic syndrome. The nephrotic phase of progressive acute (post-streptococcal) glomerulonephritis is brief if it occurs at all, because the glomerular filtration rate falls rapidly, reducing the loss of protein in the urine and relieving the oedema. A short period of well-being may follow, but a rising blood pressure and falling glomerular filtration rate lead to death from renal failure or from complications of hypertension, usually in 6 months to 2 years. Many cases of proliferative glomerulonephritis, however, present insidiously with oedema and have no demonstrable relationship to streptococcal infection. The clinical course and prognosis of these cases are extremely variable.

In membranous glomerulonephritis, hypertension occurs late in the disease and the deterioration in renal function is slow. Most patients live for 5 years and some for as long as 20 years.

In minimal lesion glomerulonephritis the blood pressure is usually normal and the glomerular filtration rate unimpaired. The oedema may be gross, and the patient severely incapacitated. Spontaneous remission can occur, however, and in the majority of cases proteinuria can be abolished, sometimes permanently, either by steroids or by cyclophosphamide. Untreated or unresponsive cases run a course of fluctuating invalidism for may years.

Investigations

1. Oedema in the nephrotic syndrome can usually be distinguished from that produced by conditions such as cardiac failure, hepatic cirrhosis or deep venous thrombosis by the presence of proteinuria. Proteinuria can complicate severe cardiac failure, however. In the nephrotic syndrome proteinuria is usually over 5.0 g per day, the serum cholesterol level is markedly raised, and the serum protein concentration is reduced, with a very low albumin level and an increased alpha 2 macroglobulin level.

2. Proteinuria due to significant renal disease should be distinguished from postural proteinuria, which requires no treatment. In postural proteinuria, urine produced when the patient is recumbent does not contain protein (p. 63).

3. The aetiology of the renal disease should be determined where possible. Glucose should be determined in blood and urine to exclude diabetes. Tests should be carried out for antinuclear factor and lupus erythematosus (LE) cells. Chronic sepsis should be sought, as should evidence of rheumatoid arthritis, Crohn's disease and ulcerative colitis. The presence of any of these raises the possibility of renal amyloid. Abundant red cell casts in the urine suggest proliferative glomerulonephritis, as does a raised anti-streptolysin O titre.

4. Renal function should be assessed by determination of the blood urea and electrolytes and the creatinine clearance. The excretion of protein in the urine should be assessed quantitatively. Differential protein clearance determinations are often helpful.

5. Management of the nephrotic syndrome is easier if the

50

precise histology of the glomerular lesions is known. For this reason, almost all nephrotic patients should have renal biopsy carried out. This point applies even in children, where renal biopsy is technically more difficult than in adults and may require a general anaesthetic.

Treatment

High protein diet. The nephrotic state is due to protein depletion. It is therefore rational to give a high protein diet, provided that there is no renal failure.

Salt restriction. The nephrotic state is aggravated by salt and water retention. It is thus logical to restrict the intake of sodium. In severe cases, this salt restriction may have to be extremely rigorous.

Diuretics. Modern diuretics are very effective, and their use often obviates the need for extreme salt restriction. (A diet containing 100 g of protein and 0.5 g of sodium is very unpalatable.)

Of the many diuretics available, bendrofluazide in a dosage of 10 mg per day is often sufficient. In more resistant cases, frusemide is the agent of choice. The usual dose of this diuretic is 40 mg per day. In some cases the amount given has to be increased to well over 200 mg per day. Massive doses of frusemide should be worked up to gradually; peripheral circulatory failure and severe potassium depletion may result from a diuresis which is too massive and too abrupt. Potassium chloride supplements should be given with both the above diuretics.

Spironolactone. This substance is an aldosterone antagonist. It inhibits sodium reabsorption in the distal tubule and promotes potassium retention. The administration of bendrofluazide or frusemide may lead to a marked increase in aldosterone production, which counteracts their diuretic action. Spironolactone is not a very effective diuretic on its own, but by antagonizing aldosterone it promotes the action of other diuretics. When spironolactone is given, serum potassium levels must be checked at frequent intervals.

Salt-poor albumin. Occasionally, all the measures described above fail to control the oedema. Intravenous salt-poor albumin may then be employed. This expands the plasma volume and promotes a diuresis. The effect is temporary, but once the oedema has been controlled, it can usually be prevented from recurring by diuretic therapy.

Steroid therapy. If the proteinuria can be abolished all the measures described above can be dispensed with. In 90 per cent of cases of minimal lesion glomerulonephritis, proteinuria can be abolished with steroid therapy. Unfortunately, the dose of steroid required is sometimes so high that Cushing's syndrome develops, and sometimes oedema recurs when steroids are withdrawn. Cyclophosphamide is often useful in patients who need intolerably large amounts of steroids, or who relapse every time steroids are withdrawn.

A few patients with SLE or proliferative glomerulonephritis also respond to steroids, but patients with membranous glomerulonephritis, renal amyloidosis and diabetic glomerulosclerosis do not.

Steroids in pharmacological doses are dangerous, and should be given only if a reasonable hope for benefit exists. This point is illustrated by the results of a trial on adult nephrosis carried out by the Medical Research Council. Despite dramatic remissions in some treated cases, the mortality in a randomly selected group of patients given steroids was slightly higher than the mortality in a group of matched controls not treated by these drugs. The moral is that patients should not be selected for steroid therapy on a random basis – hence the importance of renal biopsies and protein selectivity determinations in the management of the nephrotic syndrome.

DISORDERS PRESENTING AS THE NEPHROTIC SYNDROME

Most cases of the nephrotic syndrome are due to glomerulonephritis. Amyloidosis, diabetic nephropathy and systemic lupus have each accounted for about 6 per cent of the cases of the nephrotic syndrome seen in the Edinburgh renal unit over the past 5 years. Other conditions are mentioned mainly out of interest; they are not met with very frequently in clinical practice.

Amyloidosis

Amyloid is an eosinophilic material consisting of protein in conjunction with chondroitin sulphate, which may be deposited in a number of sites, including the kidneys. Amyloidosis may be

(1) congenital, (2) primary or (3) secondary to some other condition, such as chronic suppuration, rheumatoid arthritis or ulcerative colitis.

In primary amyloidosis, amyloid is more often found in the tongue, heart and gastro-intestinal tract than in the kidneys.

In secondary amyloidosis, which is now most frequently seen as a complication of long-standing rheumatoid arthritis, amyloid is deposited predominantly in parenchymatous organs, and the kidneys are involved in over 60 per cent of cases.

In congenital amyloidosis, amyloid is usually deposited in peripheral nerves and rarely in the kidney.

Amyloid stains characteristically with Congo red. On electron microscopy the actual structure of the protein can be made out, deposited in the basement membrane.

Renal amyloidosis tends to give rise to heavy proteinuria and the nephrotic syndrome. Diuretic therapy and salt restriction improve the oedema, but death from renal failure usually occurs within 3 years of diagnosis.

The progress of the disease may be halted if the causative condition (e.g. sepsis) can be eradicated. Cortico-steroids have no beneficial effect, and may make the condition worse. Massive doses of vitamin C are said by some authorities to be of benefit, but there is as yet little evidence that this therapy is effective.

Diabetic Nephropathy

Renal lesions are the cause of death in about 20 per cent of diabetics.

There are a number of ways in which diabetes can affect the kidneys:

1. Electron microscopy reveals some degree of *basement membrane thickening* in all diabetics.

2. Most diabetic patients sooner or later develop *diffuse glomerulosclerosis*, the main feature of which is thickening of the walls of the glomerular capillaries. This thickening varies enormously in extent from one patient to another.

3. The most characteristic renal lesions in diabetes are *Kimmelstiel-Wilson lesions.* These consist of nodular depositions of hyaline material in the periphery of glomeruli. Such lesions are frequently seen in post-mortem material, but are less often found in biopsy material, because they are patchy in distribution.

4. *Pyelonephritis.* Diabetics are more liable than non-diabetics to infections of all kinds. They are prone to both acute and chronic pyelonephritis, and severe infections can cause *renal papillary necrosis.* Necrosis of the renal papillae can also occur in diabetes in the absence of infection.

Symptomless proteinuria is very common in diabetics who have had the disease for 15 years or more. It is intermittent at first, and persistent later, but only occasionally is it severe enough to cause the nephrotic syndrome. Patients may progress to renal failure without passing through a nephrotic stage. Diabetics with severe renal involvement invariably have severe diabetic retinopathy.

Urinary tract infections can be treated with antibiotics. Other renal manifestations of diabetes are relatively unresponsive to therapy, though it is thought that careful control of the diabetic state may delay their onset. Pituitary ablation leads to improvement in the basement membrane changes, but has no effect on the vascular lesions. Steroids have no effect on diabetic glomerulosclerosis and increase the severity of the diabetes.

Systemic Lupus Erythematosus (SLE)

Systemic lupus erythematosus is a generalized disorder of connective tissue, which can produce arthritis, serious effusions, skin rashes and renal lesions as well as many other manifestations. In acute cases there is usually pyrexia associated with leucopenia. Females are affected 10 times more often than males. The blood usually gives a positive test for antinuclear factor and LE cells may be found, particularly in active stages of the disease.

Renal involvement occurs in about 50 per cent of cases of SLE, and is a frequent cause of death. The clinical picture may be that of an acute, fulminating glomerulonephritis, but is more often that of the nephrotic syndrome. The glomeruli show proliferative changes which (at least in the early stages) tend to be focal. Occasionally a single capillary will appear extremely thickened as the result of fibrinoid necrosis, resembling a loop of wire. Wire loop lesions are virtually diagnostic of SLE. In addition, there is irregular thickening of the glomerular basement membrane, and examination under the electron microscope of sections treated with osmium shows dark deposits in the basement membrane. These 'osmophilic' lesions are characteristic of

SLE, but are also seen in other renal conditions.

Early in the course of renal involvement there is often protein-uria with little impairment in renal function. At this stage, there is a good chance of reversing the renal lesions with steroid therapy. Once a degree of renal failure has developed there is little chance of such reversal. Now, however, the prognosis is so bad that steroid therapy should probably still be tried. Protein-uria will never be abolished in the advanced case, but the progress of the disease may be delayed.

Malaria

Patients with long-standing malaria frequently have large amounts of antibody to the parasite, and the immunological reaction tends to involve the glomeruli and cause the nephrotic syndrome. This is particularly likely to occur in infections due to *Plasmodium malariae.*

(Falciparum malaria can produce 'blackwater fever'. Massive haemolysis occurs and haemoglobin is excreted in the urine. This can lead to tubular necrosis and acute renal failure. Blackwater fever is not a cause of the nephrotic syndrome.)

Renal Vein Thrombosis

This may be acute and associated with severe lumbar and abdominal pain, but more often is insidious with heavy protein-uria and oedema, but little in the way of other symptoms. Renal vein thrombosis is often secondary to abdominal tumours or to other renal disorders such as amyloidosis, but about 50 per cent of cases appear to be primary. It causes renal lesions similar to those of membranous glomerulonephritis. The progress of these lesions can sometimes be arrested by anticoagulant therapy or surgical removal of the clot. The latter procedure is possible only if the clot is in a large vein.

Thrombosis of the inferior vena cava at or above the level of the renal veins produces the same effect as thrombosis of the renal veins themselves.

Nephrotic Syndrome in Infancy

In infancy the nephrotic syndrome may be due to *congenital idiopathic nephrosis,* or to *congenital syphilis.* Although both are rare, it is important to distinguish between them, because syphilitic nephrosis responds well to appropriate therapy, while congenital idiopathic nephrosis does not appear to be influenced by any form of treatment.

Other Causes of the Nephrotic Syndrome

The nephrotic syndrome may also arise from immune reaction to injections of foreign protein (e.g. as part of the syndrome known as serum sickness which may follow passive immunization with horse serum) and from hypersensitivity reactions to pollen, insect bites or a variety of drugs. Of the numerous chemicals which have been described as causing the nephrotic syndrome, troxidone (used for petit mal), penicillamine (used for Wilson's disease), and heavy metals such as gold, mercury and bismuth, are perhaps the most important. Although patients usually recover once they are removed from contact with the causative agent, 5 out of a series of 15 cases of troxidone nephropathy died of renal disease despite withdrawal of the drug.

DISORDERS PRESENTING IN OTHER WAYS

Polyarteritis Nodosa

Polyarteritis nodosa is a collagen disease which involves small or medium-sized vessels in many parts of the body. The vessel walls are acutely involved and are infiltrated with polymorphonuclear leucocytes. Polyarteritis may also involve the major branches of the renal arteries, and cause renal infarction. Involvement of the smaller vessels causes a focal proliferative glomerulonephritis, the clinical picture of which resembles that seen in acute nephritis, but the prognosis of which is much worse.

Males are affected more often than females, and the peak incidence is in the seventh decade.

The diagnosis can be confirmed by finding blod vessels showing the characteristic histological pattern in a biopsy taken from the kidney or some other affected tissue, such as muscle. Polyarteritis is treated with cortico-steroids.

Wegener's Granulomatosis

This rare disease is regarded as a variant of polyarteritis, and in addition to renal lesions identical to those seen in polyarteritis, granulomata appear in the nasal sinuses and in the lung parenchyma. This condition has a bad prognosis, but death may be delayed for a number of years if steroid therapy is started early enough.

Goodpasture's Syndrome

This rare disease is characterized by lung purpura and nephritis. Ninety per cent of patients are men. The basis of both the lung and the renal lesions appears to be immunological; it is thought that the renal glomeruli and lung alveoli share a common antigen. Most cases are rapidly fatal and as many die of their lung condition as of renal failure. Although steroids in high dosage and immuno-suppressive therapy in the form of azothiaprone have been tried, over 90 per cent of patients die within days or weeks of developing the disease.

The Haemolytic-Uraemic Syndrome

This is a hypersensitivity reaction that may occur in infants or young children as a systemic disturbance, associated with vomiting and diarrhoea, and be followed by fairly massive haemolysis with thrombocytopaenia and renal failure. The renal failure may be caused by tubular necrosis, by changes resembling those of proliferative glomerulonephritis or by both.

The hypersensitivity reaction damages blood vessels, and this is followed by intravascular coagulation. The agent causing hypersensitivity varies from case to case. In South America, a virus can be incriminated as the cause in many cases, but in Europe it is unusual for a causative agent to be identified.

The disease has a high mortality, but recent evidence suggests that a combination of steroids (which depress the immune reaction) and anticoagulants (which limit intravascular clotting) is effective in a proportion of cases.

Thrombotic Thrombocytopaenic Purpura

This extremely rare condition occurs in adults, and consists of widespread intravascular coagulation. It may involve so many red blood cells that haemolytic anaemia develops, and so many platelets that thrombocytopaenia occurs, causing severe bleeding. Acute renal failure is common, and tends to be rapidly fatal.

This condition may be the adult equivalent of haemolytic-uraemic syndrome. Treatment with steroids and anticoagulants has been tried, with encouraging results in a few isolated cases. Despite the paradox of anticoagulating patients who are already bleeding, the prognosis in untreated cases is so appalling that there is little to be lost by this course of action. Attempts to reverse the thrombocytopaenia by splenectomy have had disappointing results.

Scleroderma

In this slowly but relentlessly progressive disease, the skin becomes indurated and fibrotic lesions appear in the lungs, gastro-intestinal tract and kidneys. Contraction of the thickened and fibrotic skin can lead to gross joint deformities. The changes may be confined to the hands, but when the disease is more widespread renal involvement occurs at some stage in most patients. The characteristic renal lesion is massive thickening of the walls of the small and medium-sized arteries, which may cause proliferative changes or fibrosis in the glomeruli.

Some patients, especially those with hypertension, progress rapidly to severe renal failure, but it is more common for the renal lesions of scleroderma to progress gradually, over years or decades.

Steroids are ineffective in this condition, and the same can be said for the host of other drugs which have been tried.

The Kidney in Myeloma

Multiple myeloma is a neoplastic disease, characterized by invasion of the bone marrow and other sites by masses of abnormal plasma cells. In X-rays multiple 'punched out' translucencies are often seen in a variety of bones, and the diagnosis can usually be confirmed by bone marrow examination. The abnormal plasma cells frequently synthesize abnormal proteins. If these proteins are of high molecular weight, they will be detectable only on protein electrophoresis of serum. If they are of low molecular

58

weight, they appear in the urine as 'Bence Jones' protein. This is characteristically insoluble at 55°C, and appears as a white precipitate if urine is moderately heated; it redissolves with further heating and precipitates again as the urine cools. Bence Jones protein can give a false negative reaction with 'stick tests' for proteinuria. In cases of suspected myeloma, salicyl sulphonic acid should be used to detect proteinuria, and the nature of the protein should then be confirmed by urine electrophoresis.

Multiple myeloma can affect the kidneys by producing a high serum uric acid or a high serum calcium, by causing renal amyloidosis, or by invasion of the renal parenchyma with plasma cells. The most characteristic pathological finding in cases with severe renal involvement is, however, the presence of many casts in the renal tubules. These casts consist mainly of Bence Jones protein, and are associated with atrophy and disintegration of neighbouring tubular cells. If the casts are sufficiently numerous and widespread they cause tubular blockage and renal failure.

Dehydration increases the likelihood of cast formation, and patients should be encouraged to drink large volumes of fluid, provided that their renal function is sufficiently good to eliminate a water load. Some patients have developed catastrophic renal failure following i.v.p. examination, not because of the procedure itself, but because of the period of dehydration which precedes it. Apart from the prevention of dehydration, attempts can be made to destroy the abnormal plasma cells with X-rays or anti-mitotic drugs. This will also reduce the production of abnormal proteins and casts. Unfortunately, this therapy liberates purines from the destroyed cells and may cause secondary gout. This complication can be controlled by allopurinol.

Henoch-Schonlein Purpura

This allergic condition, which is also known as 'anaphylactoid purpura', is characterized by a purpuric rash associated with abdominal pain, joint pains and haematuria. The agent responsible for this hypersensitivity reaction varies from patient to patient and usually cannot be identified.

The renal lesions are those of proliferative glomerulonephritis, and are possibly caused by immunological mechanisms similar to those responsible for post-streptococcal acute nephritis. In

59

Henoch-Schonlein purpura, however, the lesions tend to be focal, and severely affected glomeruli lie adjacent to entirely normal ones.

The disease is much commoner in children than in adults, and in children the recovery rate is over 90 per cent. In 50 per cent of adults the renal lesions are progressive, and lead to chronic renal failure.

Cortico-steroids suppress the extra-renal manifestations of the disease, but have little effect on the glomerular lesions. In patients with progressive renal damage, immuno-suppressive agents such as azothiaprine have been tried, but there is as yet no firm evidence that they are effective.

Renal Lesions in Subacute Bacterial Endocarditis

Proteinuria and haematuria commonly occur in subacute bacterial endocarditis. At one time it was thought that multiple emboli thrown off from the infected valves caused the renal lesions, but the histological appearances are those of a focal pro-liferative glomerulonephritis, and it is now believed that an immune response to the infecting organisms causes the lesions.

Gout and the Kidneys

Primary gout is a metabolic disorder of obscure aetiology in which the blood uric acid level is moderately raised over a pro-longed period, and uric acid is deposited in various sites, including subcutaneous tissues, joint spaces and renal tissue.

Secondary gout may arise either from *increased uric acid pro-duction,* in conditions such as polycythaemia, leukaemia or myeloma, or from *decreased uric acid excretion,* as in chronic renal failure. In myeloproliferative disorders, radiotherapy or cytotoxic drugs can lead to massive breakdown of cells, and a massive rise in the plasma uric acid level. Diuretics such as chlorothiazide or frusemide interfere with tubular secretion of uric acid, and can precipitate gout in patients with a moderately elevated uric acid level.

Renal lesions

Urates are deposited in the interstitial spaces of the kidneys, between the tubules. They cause an inflammatory reaction known as 'interstitial nephritis', with degeneration of adjacent tubular cells.

'Nephrosclerosis', which is the term given to the vascular changes seen in the kidneys of patients with long-standing hypertension, may occur in gout, even when the blood pressure is normal.

When the renal excretion of uric acid is high, uric acid stones may form, particularly in acid urine. Uric acid can also be precipitated within the renal tubules, and cause tubular obstruction. Finally, appearances similar to those seen in chronic glomerulonephritis may occur, with basement membrane thickening and endothelial cell proliferation.

If the serum uric acid level is very high the danger of acute renal failure from tubular obstruction may be minimized by combining a high fluid intake with the administration of sodium bicarbonate, to ensure a high flow of alkaline urine.

If the uric acid serum level is moderately high, uricosuric agents such as probenecid, which interfere with tubular reabsorption of uric acid, minimize deposition of uric acid in tissues, but will not prevent the production of uric acid stones because they increase uric acid excretion. If renal function is already impaired, or if stones form, allopurinol is of benefit. Allopurinol interferes with the enzyme xanthine oxidase, and decreases uric acid production so that xanthine and hypoxanthine, instead of uric acid, are excreted in the urine. Xanthine stones have not as yet been reported following the use of allopurinol.

Renal Lesions in Leukaemia

The kidneys may be infiltrated by leukaemic cells, or damaged by the increased uric acid production associated with the rapid turnover of white blood cells. Leukaemic patients have a reduced resistance to infection, and may develop pyelonephritis.

Sickle Cell Anaemia

This is a form of congenital haemolytic anaemia which occurs in people of African descent. The red blood cells contain an abnormal haemoglobin, haemoglobin S, have a sickle-shaped appearance, and are fragile and haemolyse.

Patients with sickle cell disease frequently have defective renal concentrating mechanisms, and it has been suggested that the red cells become even more sickle-shaped in the hypertonic renal medulla and impair medullary circulation. Massive renal infarction, especially of the medulla, can occur in sickle cell disease, possibly on the basis of a similar mechanism.

Sarcoidosis

Although the kidneys may be involved by sarcoid granulomata, they are more often damaged by the hypercalcaemia which sarcoid causes. Treatment is with cortico-steroids.

Pregnancy and the Kidney

The ureters and the renal pelvis are always dilated during and for some months after pregnancy, and *pyelonephritis* is a frequent complication.

Acute tubular necrosis may occur in such complications of pregnancy as septic abortion, ruptured ectopic gestation, concealed accidental haemorrhage and post-partum haemorrhage.

The condition specific to pregnancy is *pre-eclamptic toxaemia.*

Pre-eclamptic toxaemia, which occurs only during pregnancy, consists of hypertension, oedema and proteinuria. The cells of the glomeruli become oedematous and interfere with the circulation through the glomerular capillaries. Fibrin is deposited in the glomeruli, especially between the endothelial cells and the basement membrane.

Although pre-eclampsia may cause severe hypertension, massive oedema, renal failure and fits, if salt intake is controlled and hypertension adequately treated, an unfavourable outcome — for the mother, at any rate — is rare, because rapid spontaneous recovery usually follows delivery.

Phenacetin Nephritis

Swiss watchmakers get headaches which they attribute to eye strain and treat with phenacetin. In 1950 it was noted that these same Swiss watchmakers tended to die of renal failure at a relatively early age. The renal lesions were similar to those seen in pyelonephritis, but were most marked in the renal interstitium.

There was chronic interstitial inflammation (especially of the cortico-medullary junction), associated with degeneration of tubular cells, and sometimes with necrosis of the renal papillae.

Although phenacetin addicts are more liable to renal infection than other people, in many such patients there is no evidence of bacterial invasion, and the lesions are attributed to phenacetin or to analgesic mixtures which contain phenacetin. Many writers refer to the condition as 'analgesic nephropathy' rather than phenacetin nephropathy.

Except in advanced cases, cessation of analgesic intake usually leads to considerable improvement in renal function.

Postural Proteinuria

Postural proteinuria typically occurs in thin young men, and disappears as they grow older and become fatter. Protein appears in the urine when the subject is standing, and disappears from the urine when the subject lies down. It seems that the liver is relatively mobile in thin young subjects, and is able to rotate to compress the inferior vena cava when they are in the erect posture. This produces back pressure in the renal veins and the renal lymphatics.

On light microscopy renal biopsy reveals no abnormality in patients with postural proteinuria. On electron microscopy glomerular changes can be seen, but their importance is difficult to assess, since there is indirect evidence that the protein in postural proteinuria is not of glomerular origin.

Postural proteinuria is a benign condition which does not progress to renal failure, and to distinguish it from other causes of proteinuria is important. The patient remains in an erect, lordotic posture for an hour, and urine passed at the end of this period is tested for protein. The patient then lies supine for 3 hours. Urine is passed after an hour and discarded, and again at the end of the period of recumbency.

If the specimen produced in the erect position contains a significant amount of protein and the specimen produced in the supine position contains no protein the patient has postural proteinuria.

FURTHER READING

Berlyne, G. M. (1967). Renal involvement in the collagen diseases. Renal involvement in other systemic diseases. In *Renal Disease,* 2nd ed. Ed. Black, D. A. K. Oxford: Blackwell.

Kassirer, J. P. & Schwartz, W. B. (1961). Acute glomerulonephritis. *New Engl. J. Med.,* **256,** 686.

Robson, J. S. (1967). The nephrotic syndrome. In *Renal Disease,* 2nd ed. Ed. Black, D. A. K. Oxford: Blackwell.

Chapter 4

RENAL FAILURE

ACUTE RENAL FAILURE

Acute renal failure is a sudden and severe reduction in renal function which causes retention of waste products and other serious defects in the regulation of the body's internal environment. It is usually associated with oliguria (i.e. a reduction in urine volume to 400 ml per day or less) but it can occur when the urinary output is normal, or even when it is increased. The causes of acute renal failure may be *pre-renal, renal* or *post-renal* in origin.

Pre-renal acute renal failure
Pre-renal acute renal failure is caused by impairment in renal perfusion. A reduced blood flow to the kidney lowers the glomerular filtration rate, and filtration ceases altogether if the pressure in the renal artery falls below 50 mm Hg. Impaired perfusion may result from a low blood volume and be produced by loss of blood, of plasma, or of fluid and electrolytes. It can also occur in conditions such as myocardial infarction, pulmonary embolism and septicaemic shock, where the blood pressure can fall catastrophically despite a normal blood volume (Table 1).

There is often little correlation between renal perfusion and the blood pressure as measured in the brachial artery. A cold and clammy patient with a systolic pressure measuring 100 mm Hg in the arm may have a complete shut-down of the renal circulation, while a patient with pink and warm extremities and a systolic brachial pressure of 70 mm Hg may have a perfectly adequate glomerular blood flow.

In most cases of impaired renal function due to hypotension or hypovolaemia, renal function can be restored simply by restoring the blood pressure and blood volume to normal. If the impairment in renal perfusion is allowed to persist, however, acute tubular necrosis or (less often) renal cortical necrosis will occur.

Table 1 Pre-renal causes of acute renal failure

A. *Impaired Renal Perfusion due to Lowered Blood Volume*

1. *Loss of Blood*
    (a) Trauma causing loss of blood to the exterior.
    (b) Haemorrhage to the gastro-intestinal tract – from varices, peptic ulcer, etc.
    (c) Haemorrhage complicating pregnancy and childbirth. (Ruptured ectopic gestation, placenta praevia, concealed accidental haemorrhage, etc.)
    (d) Haemorrhage into soft tissues – after crush injuries to muscle; following fracture of femoral shaft, etc.
    (e) Into body cavities – as in splenic rupture.

2. *Loss of Plasma*
    (a) From the body surface, following severe and extensive burns.
    (b) Into the gastro-intestinal tract (along with some blood) in infarction of the bowel.
    (c) Into the peritoneal cavity (with blood and ECF in variable proportions) following acute pancreatitis or severe peritonitis.

3. *Loss of Water and Electrolytes*
    (a) From the gastro-intestinal tract – in paralytic ileus.
        intestinal obstruction.
        severe vomiting of whatever cause.
        severe diarrhoea.
    (b) From the kidneys – in uncontrolled diabetes or in Addison's disease.
    (c) From the skin – profuse sweating, with inadequate or inappropriate replacement (as in 'heat stroke').
    (d) From fistulae – draining structures such as the gall bladder.

B. *Factors Impairing Renal Perfusion Without Reduction of Blood Volume*

1. *Myocardial Infarction.*
2. *Massive Pulmonary Embolism.*
3. *Septicaemic Shock.*

All the above factors may also cause renal uraemia, since prolonged impairment of renal perfusion will cause acute tubular necrosis or renal cortical necrosis.

The above are *examples* of situations in which renal failure may occur; the list is not a comprehensive one.

Renal causes of acute renal failure

In this situation impairment of renal function is produced or maintained by structural damage to the kidneys themselves.

Any of the causes of pre-renal acute renal failure can lead either to acute tubular necrosis (which is reversible) or to the more sinister renal cortical necrosis (which is not). Acute tubular necrosis can also arise as the result of nephrotoxic agents (p. 68).

Many of the conditions discussed in Chapter 3 can present acutely, with severe and abrupt reduction in renal function. Acute glomerulonephritis, malignant hypertension and polyarteritis nodosa in particular may present from the outset as severe oliguria with a rapidly climbing blood urea. If a patient with acute renal failure has no history of hypotension or hypovolaemia, primary renal disease should be suspected.

Chronic renal disease may progress insidiously to produce a major reduction in renal function, but little in the way of symptoms. If the renal reserve is severely reduced, an intercurrent infection (by increasing urea production) or a gastro-intestinal upset (by causing dehydration) may precipitate a severe degree of uraemia, and in this way chronic renal disease may present acutely. Acute-on-chronic renal failure is suggested by the presence of a moderately severe normocytic anaemia and by a history of ill-health going back over several months. Plain X-rays of the abdomen may be useful in diagnosis, as they may show the outlines of scarred and contracted kidneys.

Post-renal acute renal failure

Obstruction in the urinary tract causes back pressure. Back pressure reduces glomerular filtration and may even cause it to cease entirely. The causes of obstruction in the urinary tract are dealt with in Chapter 7. Relief of the obstruction restores renal function, unless back pressure and infection have led to the destruction of a considerable amount of renal parenchyma.

Complete anuria is suggestive of obstruction, as are periods of anuria alternating with periods of polyuria. Abdominal pain, especially if it has the characteristics of renal colic, is also suggestive of a block to the free passage of urine. Obstruction causing renal failure is obviously more common in patients who possess only one functioning kidney than in patients with two.

Early diagnosis and early treatment are vitally important in renal failure due to post-renal causes. For this reason it is essential to exclude the presence of obstruction in all cases where the cause of impaired renal function is not obvious. In the early stages of obstruction, before any structural damage to the kidney has occurred, an ^{131}I Hippuran renogram will give a characteristic pattern. The only way to be certain whether or not obstruction is present, however, is to carry out cystoscopy and ureteric catheterization.

Acute Tubular Necrosis

Acute tubular necrosis is the commonest and most important cause of acute renal failure. It is one of the relatively few conditions in medicine where early diagnosis and correct management can make all the difference between cure and death. Any doctor in any clinical field can find himself with a case of acute tubular necrosis on his hands. The condition may be treated by a renal physician, but the early diagnosis must be made by the surgeon, the obstetrician or the paediatrician – and on occasion by the practitioner in skins, eyes or geriatrics.

Aetiology

Acute tubular necrosis may arise in any situation where there is hypovolaemia or hypotension (Table 1).

It can also be produced by *nephrotoxic substances.* Agents with nephrotoxic effects are numerous; they can be classified under three headings:

1. *Exogenous chemicals,* e.g. heavy metals, phenols, carbon tetrachloride, chlorate, ethylene glycol, sulphonamides.

2. *Bacterial toxins* – particularly those released in the course of Gram-negative septicaemias.

3. *Endogenous substances in excess,* e.g. free circulating haemoglobin, porphyrins, bilirubin.

Acute tubular necrosis is rare in mild hypotension, uncomplicated jaundice or transient bacteraemia. If a patient with obstructive jaundice develops a bacteraemia with a moderate fall in blood pressure, however, acute tubular necrosis is likely to occur. Nephrotoxic agents appear to potentiate the damage caused to tubular cells by impaired renal perfusion.

A summary of some of the factors which can produce tubular necrosis is given in Table 2.

Pathology

At first sight the glomeruli appear relatively normal. Vasoconstriction leads to stasis in the renal vessels, however, and on careful examination 'sludging' of cells and platelets, along with fibrin deposition, is seen in many small vessels, including the glomerular capillaries.

Differences exist between the tubular lesions produced by renal ischaemia and those produced by nephrotoxic substances.

68

Many nephrotoxins are secreted by the cells of the proximal tubule, and their concentration in these cells tends to be much greater than their concentration anywhere else. Nephrotoxins cause death of proximal tubular cells, causing damage to a considerable length of the proximal tubule, and affecting all proximal tubules more or less equally. The tubular basement membrane remains intact.

Table 2 Genesis of acute tubular necrosis

Hypotension due to:
  Blood loss
  Loss of plasma
  Fluid and electrolyte depletion
  Cardiogenic shock
  Septicaemic shock   *reduces renal blood flow*

Reduced renal blood flow
  1. Lowers the glomerular filtration
      rate and   *causes pre-renal uraemia*
  2. Interferes with the blood supply of
      the kidneys and   *causes acute tubular necrosis*
                                       (rarely, *renal cortical necrosis*)

Nephrotoxic substances
(Exogenous chemicals, bacterial
toxins, certain endogenous
substances)
  1. Damage tubular cells and are a
      direct cause of   *acute tubular necrosis*
  2. Cause renal vasoconstriction or
      renal vascular necrosis
                  and
      by interfering with renal perfusion
      are an indirect cause of   *acute tubular necrosis*

Ischaemic lesions are patchily distributed, and may occur at any site in the nephron. They affect a relatively short segment of tubule, but in this segment there is rupture of the tubular basement membrane in addition to death of the cells (Fig. 16).

A mixed picture is not uncommon, as many nephrotoxins in addition to damaging the tubules directly, also produce renal ischaemia.

Tubular necrosis is associated with a severe reduction in *glomerular* filtration. The impaired glomerular function can be explained as follows.

1. Fibrin deposition in the glomerular arterioles reduces filtration pressure, while sludging of cells and platelets in the glomerular capillaries causes further interference with filtration.

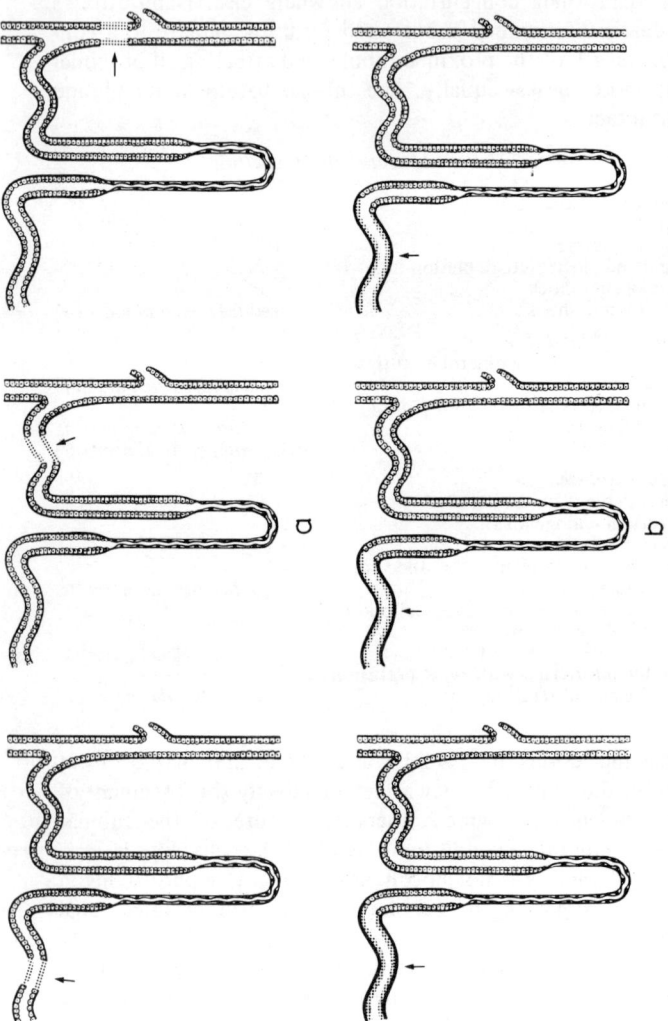

Fig. 16. The lesions of acute tubular necrosis due to (a) ischaemia and (b) nephrotoxins. Ischaemic lesions are patchily distributed and affect the entire thickness of the tubule, including the tubular basement membrane. Lesions caused by nephrotoxins affect the proximal tubule, all proximal tubules being affected to approximately the same extent. There is death of tubular cells, but the tubular basement membrane remains intact.

2. The tubules become blocked by swollen tubular cells and by necrotic cell debris within the tubular lumen.

Clinical features

The clinical picture of acute tubular necrosis is often dominated by the surgical, medical or obstetrical calamity causing it. The manifestations also depend on the severity of the biochemical disturbance and the rate at which the disturbance has developed. Most illnesses increase the breakdown of body protein. In severe infections, major trauma to soft tissues, or severe burns the rate of breakdown of body protein may be very high indeed. Acute tubular necrosis often occurs in hypercatabolic situations where the blood urea tends to rise at a rate of 100 mg per cent per day, or more. In the absence of infection and trauma, with adequate calories and restriction of dietary protein, the blood urea may rise by as little as 25 mg per cent per day, even in total anuria. The severely catabolic patient presents a much more difficult problem in management than the patient in whom biochemical abnormalities develop gradually.

A raised blood urea level is a constant finding in patients with severe renal failure. Patients with a high blood urea have a number of clinical features which are described as uraemic manifestations, although there is little to suggest that these manifestations are caused by urea.

Uraemic manifestations. Salivation is decreased, and the patient complains of a dry mouth. There is a tendency for mouth ulceration to occur, with complications such as moniliasis and parotitis.

Anorexia, nausea and vomiting may occur. The reduced food intake which results often produces constipation, but in severe uraemia ulcers may appear at virtually any point in the gastrointestinal tract, and give rise to a severe, often bloody, diarrhoea.

A bleeding tendency is common. This is ascribed to impaired platelet *function*; it can occur in the presence of a normal platelet count. Correction of the uraemia (e.g. by dialysis) usually corrects this bleeding tendency.

Mental disturbances are common. Uraemic patients are drowsy and lethargic, and with a steadily rising blood urea, coma eventually occurs. Psychiatric disturbances are often seen. These may range from mild confusion and disorientation to mania, depression or paranoid delusions.

There is increased neuromuscular excitability, with muscle twitching and hiccough, and on occasion grand mal seizures.

Salt and water overload can occur very easily on account of the reduced urinary output, and lead to oedema, hypertension and pulmonary oedema. In renal failure the kidneys are unable to excrete hydrogen ions, and in hypercatabolism the acid load is increased as well as the nitrogen load. A severe metabolic acidosis is common in renal failure, and this leads to hyperventilation. In acidosis, hydrogen ions enter cells, displacing potassium ions. Potassium is also added to the extracellular fluid from the breakdown of cells. A high serum potassium may lead to paraesthesia followed by muscle weakness, but the first and only manifestation may be cardiac arrest. Potassium intoxication is discussed further on p. 82. Uraemic patients are extremely susceptible to infection, and once an infection has become established eradication is difficult while the uraemia persists.

Prolonged uraemia is associated with pericarditis, neuropathy and metabolic bone disease. These features take some time to develop and are rarely seen in acute renal failure. They are discussed on pp. 78–82.

One fortunate thing about acute tubular necrosis is that recovery of renal function always occurs, provided the patient survives. The initial *oliguric phase* is replaced after a few days or a few weeks by a *diuretic phase* in which the urine volume is greater than normal, sometimes by a considerable amount. The high urine volume of the diuretic phase is due partly to the osmotic diuresis produced by the high blood urea, and partly to the impaired ability of the recovering tubules to conserve filtered salts and water. During the diuretic phase patients can become depleted of potassium, sodium and water, and if losses in the urine are not made good, death may complicate diuresis.

Figure 17 shows the clinical course of a reasonably typical case of tubular necrosis.

Management

The cause of the acute renal failure must be found and corrected. Fluid deficits should be made good, promptly. The osmolality and the urine urea concentration should be checked; if the osmotic concentration is over 500 m.osm/kg and the urea content over 1.0 g per cent, tubular necrosis may not be established, and it is worth trying to induce a diuresis by giving 200 ml of 20 per cent mannitol intravenously. If this has no effect no attempt should be made to push fluids after the patient has become normally hydrated. It is sometimes difficult to judge whether or not a patient's blood volume has been fully expanded, and in this situation it is often useful to pass an intravenous

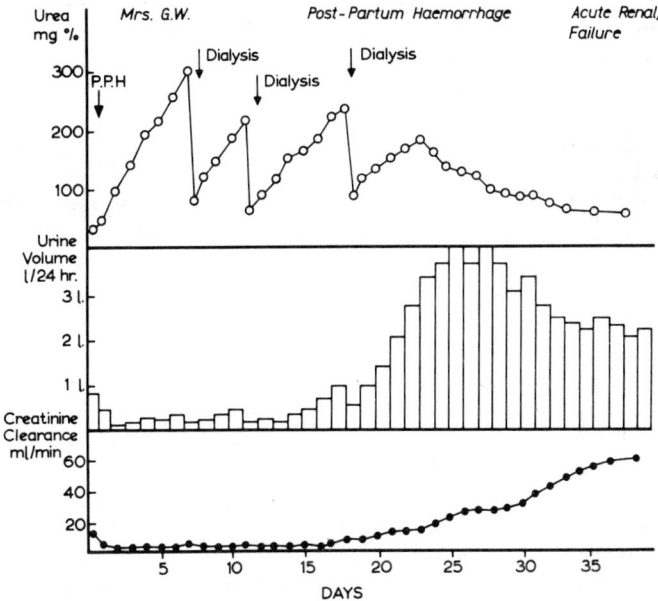

Fig. 17. The course of a case of acute tubular necrosis, which occurred following post-partum haemorrhage. The oliguric phase lasted about three weeks, and three dialyses were required during this period. The diuretic phase then followed, with urine volumes approaching 4 litres daily. By 37 days the blood urea and urine volume had returned to normal and the creatinine clearance had risen to 60 ml per minute. The rate of rise of blood urea in this patient (40 mg per 100 ml per day during the oliguric phase) was considerably less than that seen in severely infected or traumatized cases.

catheter into the superior vena cava or right atrium to measure the central venous pressure. Fluids should be given until the central venous pressure is in the region of plus 2.0 cm of water. In septicaemic shock, the blood volume may be normal, but hypotension may be present because of inappropriate vasodilatation, particularly in the splanchnic vessels. The blood pressure can be corrected by infusing plasma or blood, monitoring the infusion by the central venous pressure. If hypotension is due to cardiac failure, digoxin should be given. The initial digitalizing dose is approximately the same as that required by patients without renal failure, but the maintenance dose is much smaller, being as a rule 0.25 mg of digoxin 3 or 4 times a week.

In every case of acute renal failure, a careful search for infection should be made, cultures being taken of blood, urine, and sputum, and from any wounds that may be present. Any infection found should be treated promptly and vigorously, but prophylactic antibiotics should not be given, as these predispose to superinfection by resistant organisms. Patients with acute tubular necrosis are very susceptible to infection, and every effort should be made to prevent them coming in contact with the dangerous cross infections that abound in hospitals.

If obstructive jaundice is present, as with a stone in the common bile duct, the obstruction must be dealt with surgically as a matter of urgency, though a pre-operative dialysis may be required to avert a metabolic death on the operating table.

Control of the renal failure can be achieved in two ways. If the patient is in fairly good condition, and the blood urea is rising relatively slowly, it is reasonable to manage him conservatively, at least for the first few days. Once the fluid and electrolyte deficit has been corrected the daily fluid intake should be reduced to 500 ml more than the urinary ouput of the previous day. The patient should be weighed daily as a check on fluid balance; if the weight is not tending to fall gradually, fluid intake is excessive. In severe oliguria, virtually no sodium and potassium are being lost in the urine. None should therefore be given in the diet. The protein content of the diet should be about 20 g per day, and over 1,000 calories should be given daily, to reduce the breakdown of body protein for energy.

In hypercatabolic cases, conservative management is doomed to failure. The only hope of survival lies in dialysis. The aim should be to dialyse early enough and often enough to prevent the development of uraemic manifestations. Adequately dialysed patients with tubular necrosis do not develop a bleeding tendency, are not confused and are in relatively slight danger of death from potassium intoxication – though potassium can on occasion rise dangerously between dialyses. The protein content of the diet need not be restricted, and as a result the gross emaciation which used to be a feature of a prolonged siege in this condition need

74

not occur. If the blood urea is prevented from rising above 200–250 mg per cent resistance to infection is reasonably well maintained.

With this approach to the treatment of tubular necrosis, provided the precipitating illness is responsive to treatment, patients should remain well-nourished and fit despite a prolonged period of oliguria. Patients with acute tubular necrosis still die of the diseases which produced the renal failure, but none should die of uraemia.

The management of the diuretic phase requires great care. There is a tendency for surveillance to become casual once urine production returns, yet occasionally patients still die with their urine production in full flood. During the diuretic phase, sodium and potassium supplements must be given – often in amounts of over 10 g of NaCl and 10 g of KC1 daily. Fluid intake, of course, must also be increased. The serum sodium and potassium must be carefully monitored during the diuretic phase, as must the blood pressure and the state of hydration of the patient.

The time of onset of the diuretic phase in acute tubular necrosis varies a great deal; it usually occurs 10 to 14 days after the onset of oliguria. If there is still no sign of a diuresis after 3 to 4 weeks, the possibility of renal cortical necrosis, or of some primary renal condition, such as a fulminant glomerulonephritis, must be considered. Renal biopsy should be considered if a diuresis has not occurred by the end of the fourth week.

Renal Cortical Necrosis

This condition occurs in the same clinical context as acute tubular necrosis, and the list of causes for tubular necrosis can be applied almost without modification to cortical necrosis. It is a rare disease in comparison with acute tubular necrosis, accounting for between 2 and 5 per cent of cases of acute renal failure. It is encountered in obstetric patients with acute renal failure more often than in other clinical contexts, and concealed accidental haemorrhage in particular seems to produce cortical necrosis more frequently than other conditions causing renal failure.

The clinical features of cortical necrosis differ from those of tubular necrosis only in the fact that renal function does not recover at the end of a 2- to 6-week period. Diagnosis depends on the appearance on renal biopsy or at post mortem. There is

75

ischaemic necrosis of the entire cortex apart from a small rim immediately beneath the renal capsule; the medulla is spared. If the patient is kept alive by dialysis for a number of weeks, calcification of the necrotic cortex frequently occurs.

The initial treatment is as for acute tubular necrosis. Once renal failure has been present for 4 or more weeks, the presence of cortical necrosis should be suspected, and a renal biopsy carried out as soon as the patient's condition permits. Once the diagnosis is established, preparations should be made either for long-term dialysis or for renal transplantation — provided that facilities are available and the patient is suitable for these forms of therapy.

CHRONIC RENAL FAILURE

In chronic renal failure a gradual falling off in renal function causes retention of waste products in the body, together with other deficiencies in the regulation of the internal environment. Because the impairment of kidney function occurs gradually and the uraemic state is more prolonged than that encountered in acute renal failure, the overall clinical picture is different in some respects. Renal anaemia, uraemic pericarditis, metabolic bone disease and uraemic neuropathy occur rarely in acute renal failure, but are seen relatively often in chronic renal failure — always provided that the patient survives long enough for these features to develop.

Aetiology
Chronic renal failure can arise from most of the disorders of renal parenchyma discussed in Chapter 3, and also from many of the causes of obstruction outlined in Chapter 7. Glomerulonephritis, malignant hypertension and chronic pyelonephritis between them account for more than 50 per cent of the cases of chronic renal failure, while congenital lesions — such as polycystic kidneys, hypoplastic kidneys or obstructive lesions of the urinary tract — are responsible for between 15 and 20 per cent.

Clinical features
The clinical course of the disease depends a great deal on whether or not severe hypertension is a complicating factor.

Hypertension causes renal damage (in addition to being produced by it) and when it is severe, renal failure progresses rapidly with the patient dying of uraemia or of cardiovascular complications after a relatively short illness. If hypertension is absent, or can be readily controlled, the patient may live for years despite severe impairment of renal function.

Although urea itself does not appear to be a particularly toxic substance, there is a fairly good correlation between the severity of the metabolic imbalance and the blood urea level. It is rare for patients to be ill from uraemia with blood urea levels of under 150 mg per cent; it is usual for the patient to have uraemic symptoms if the blood urea level is over 250 mg per cent for any length of time. The relationship between the blood urea level and the glomerular filtration rate is shown in Figure 18. It will be seen from this diagram that an abnormally large load of nitrogenous waste products (whether derived from a high protein diet or from increased catabolism of body protein) is as important in elevating the blood urea level as the degree of impairment in renal function.

Patients with blood urea levels of 100–150 mg per cent usually have nocturia because they cannot produce a

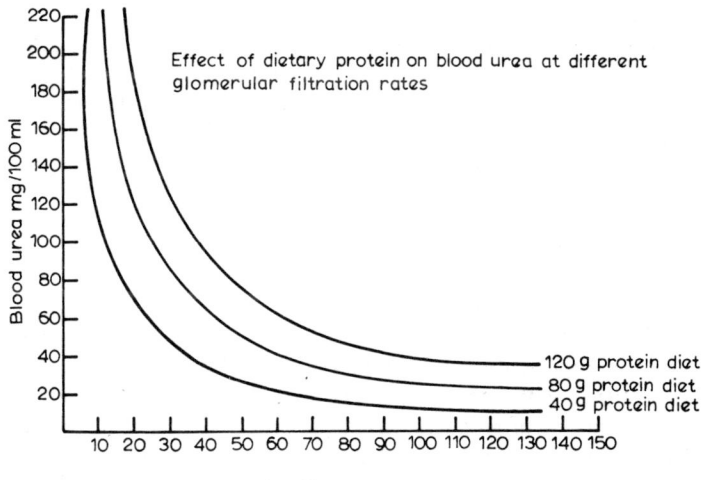

Fig. 18 The effect of variation in dietary protein intake on the blood urea at various glomerular filtration rates.

concentrated urine. They may also have a true polyuria, due to the osmotic diuresis produced by the large amount of urea filtered through each of the few surviving nephrons.

Patients with blood urea levels of 200 mg per cent or over usually have many of the features of the *uraemic syndrome.*

Pigmentation. Normal urine contains a variety of pigments and has a yellowish-brown appearance. In renal failure, these pigments are retained in the body, imparting a bronzed appearance to the skin which may be readily mistaken for a healthy sun-tan. Because of this most uraemic patients look less anaemic than they are.

Pruritis. Some uraemic patients complain of almost unbearable itching in the skin. A number of retained metabolic products may be responsible; but in some cases pruritis appears to be due to subcutaneous deposition of calcium phosphate.

Petechiae. The bleeding tendency which occurs in renal failure has already been discussed, as have the gastro-intestinal and cerebral features of the uraemic syndrome (p. 71).

Renal anaemia

Anaemia in chronic renal failure may be due in part to the bleeding tendency which exists in uraemia. Blood loss, particularly from the gastro-intestinal tract, is common. In patients with severe uraemia, there is also a degree of haemolysis. Patients who lack functioning kidneys, however, are uniformly anaemic even when they are maintained biochemically normal by haemodialysis, and when no bleeding tendency is apparent. The anaemia is normochromic and normocytic, and the bone marrow appears normal. It is thought that this anaemia is due to lack of the hormone erythropoietin.

The evidence for the production by the kidneys of a humoral agent of importance in erythropoiesis is as follows.

Patients with renal carcinoma, polycystic kidneys or simple renal cysts are often polycythaemic. Renal polycythaemia (unlike polycythaemia vera) affects the red cells series only, and the spleen is rarely enlarged. The active principle, erythropoietin, appears to be a protein with a molecular weight of about 30,000. It is rapidly inactivated when it is stored or processed; for this

78

reason it has not as yet been possible to characterize erythropoietin precisely.

Animals subjected to bilateral nephrectomy and kept biochemically normal by peritoneal dialysis become rapidly anaemic.

Animals with ureters transplanted into the inferior vena cava do not become anaemic, even if severe uraemia is allowed to develop. This indicates that normal renal tissue — rather than normal renal function — is essential for the normal production of red blood cells.

Erythropoietin is not available for therapeutic use and the only treatment for renal anaemia — other than kidney transplantation — is transfusion. Even in the absence of renal tissue, some red cell production continues, and the haemoglobin level can usually be kept between 40 and 55 per cent without transfusion. It is occasionally essential to transfuse patients with renal anaemia, but giving blood tends to depress the erythropoiesis already present. Multiple transfusions carry a high risk of transfusion reactions and/or viral hepatitis. In patients with depressed but useful renal function, raising the haematocrit leads to a fall in glomerular filtration rate. There is also the very real risk of precipitating cardiac failure.

For a variety of reasons, therefore, patients with renal anaemia should be transfused as infrequently as their clinical condition will allow.

Uraemic neuropathy

Loss of tendon jerks and slowing of nerve conduction velocities can often be demonstrated in chronic renal failure. Clinically important changes in peripheral nerves, however, occur only in patients with renal failure of long standing. In the early days of intermittent dialysis disabling neuropathy became distressingly common, because patients were as a rule dialysed at infrequent intervals, remaining alive but uraemic for prolonged periods of time. Now that dialysis in chronic renal failure is being carried out more intensively, severe neuropathy is rarer.

Demyelination and degeneration occur in the axis cylinders of peripheral nerves. The longest nerves are the most severely affected. The legs are involved much more often than the arms, and the changes occur distally rather than proximally. Hyperaemia of the lower limbs may occur in association with hyperalgesia to produce what is termed the 'burning feet syndrome'.

Later sensory loss develops along with motor weakness. A bilateral foot drop is characteristic; wrist drop is much less common.

The sensory changes of uraemic neuropathy usually improve rapidly once the patient is adequately dialysed. Loss of motor power, however, is much more intractable, and may not recover for years – or at all.

Uraemic pericarditis

Pericarditis occurs frequently in severe and prolonged uraemia. Before the advent of dialysis therapy it was regarded as a harbinger of doom; death was usual within a few days of pericarditis being detected. The patient usually complains of left-sided pleuritic pain, and this pain has some postural characteristics – sometimes, for example, being less severe when the patient bends forwards. The diagnosis is confirmed by hearing a pericardial friction rub, and the contour of the heart on chest X-ray is also helpful in diagnosis. The electrocardiograph is usually abnormal, but the abnormalities are often non-specific.

With dialysis therapy it is now possible to resuscitate patients even when they have progressed to pericarditis. Until the pericarditis has resolved, however, there is constant danger of bleeding into the inflamed pericardial sac, with cardiac tamponade and sudden death. The administration of heparin for dialysis purposes may precipitate this mode of demise. Patients with chronic renal failure should be started on dialysis therapy before they develop pericarditis, if this is at all possible.

Uraemic osteodystrophy

All patients with uraemia have disordered calcium and phosphate metabolism, but changes in bone are relatively slow to develop. In adults uraemic osteodystrophy is largely confined to those patients in whom renal failure has been present for a number of years. In children, osteodystrophy is rather more common, appearing earlier in the course of the disease. This is because a growing child lays down new bone more rapidly than an adult.

Absorption of calcium from the gut is severely impaired in uraemia – probably because there is resistance to the actions of vitamin D. Osteoblasts continue to manufacture osteoid tissue (the framework on which calcium salts are laid down to produce

80

bone) but because of the low serum calcium level and the ineffective action of vitamin D, mineralization of this framework is defective. Seams of osteoid tissue eventually appear in place of normal bone, giving rise to osteomalacia in adults and renal rickets in children. Osteoid is structurally weak, and bone deformities and pathological fractures occur.

A low serum calcium level stimulates the parathyroid glands to secrete parathormone. All patients with chronic renal failure have abnormally high serum levels of parathormone, but in many cases the serum calcium levels remain low and the bone changes of hyperparathyroidism fail to appear – suggesting that in these cases the hormone has little biological activity. In other patients, however, the hormone is effective. Serum calcium levels rise towards normal and (if the patient survives) the bone lesions of parathyroid overactivity make their appearance. Parathormone increases the activity of the osteoclasts, breaking down bone and releasing calcium into the circulation. The osteoclastic activity is maximal under the periosteum of bone and along the margins of the Haversian canals. The resorbed bone is replaced by fibrous tissue and by cysts, and the name given to the resulting bone lesions is osteitis fibrosa cystica.

In chronic renal failure, the picture is not simply one of reduced bone mineralization, but also one of erratic bone formation. In some patients, the total bulk of the skeleton is actually increased. A local increase in bone thickness appears on X-ray as a region of increased bone density, and this radiological appearance is referred to as osteosclerosis. An individual patient with metabolic bone disease resulting from renal failure may have osteomalacia, osteitis fibrosa cystica, osteosclerosis or a combination of all three conditions.

The treatment of renal osteodystrophy is complex, and will not be discussed in detail. The basic principle is to give vitamin D in high dosage. This improves absorption of calcium from the gut, and the serum calcium level rises. Because of the high serum phosphate levels which are found in patients with renal failure, a rise in serum calcium levels tends to produce deposition of calcium phosphate in soft tissues. The calcium level should not be permitted to rise to abnormal heights. If metastatic calcification occurs, aluminium hydroxide can be given. This binds phosphate in the bowel, and lowers its serum concentration.

In some patients the hypertrophied parathyroid glands

become autonomous, and continue to produce parathormone in excess even when the serum calcium levels have returned to normal. In these patients the serum calcium level rises to above normal levels. This situation is sometimes referred to as tertiary hyperparathyroidism. It is treated by excision of most of the hypertrophied parathyroid tissue.

Tetany

A low serum calcium level increases neuromuscular irritability, and can lead to tetany and to convulsions. Tetany is less common in chronic renal failure than might be expected, because most patients have a degree of acidosis and this counteracts the effects of the low serum calcium. If a hypocalcaemic, acidotic patient has his acidosis corrected by a sudden infusion of bicarbonate, however, tetany is very likely to occur. Tetany can be avoided by correcting acidosis gradually rather than rapidly, and treated by giving 20 ml of 10 per cent calcium gluconate intravenously, over a period of about 2 minutes. The effect of calcium injection is temporary, and if tetany is a persistent or recurrent problem, or if convulsions occur which can be attributed to hypocalcaemia, the serum calcium level can be raised more definitively by giving vitamin D in large doses.

Potassium intoxication

Normal kidneys can compensate promptly for a rise in the serum potassium concentration. In renal failure, elimination of excess potassium is sluggish, and there is a risk of hyperkalaemia.

The electrical activity of nervous and muscular tissue depends on the ratio between the potassium concentration within the cells and the concentration in the extracellular compartment. Most of the potassium in the body is intracellular, and relatively small changes in the amount of extracellular potassium produce large changes in the serum potassium concentration and in the intracellular/extracellular concentration ratio. The normal serum potassium concentration is 3.5 to 5.0 mEq/1. At serum levels of 7.5 to 8.0 mEq/1 cardiac arrest may be imminent. The serum potassium may rise as the result of any of the following:

1. A high potassium intake.
2. Reduced renal function.
3. A systemic acidosis. (Hydrogen ions are positively charged, and when they enter cells, they displace potassium ions.)

82

4. Destruction of body cells. Dead cells release the potassium which they contain into the extracellular fluid. Blood in the gut or elsewhere in the body will break down to release potassium into the body.

5. Interference with carbohydrate metabolism. When glucose enters cells, it carries potassium in with it. When carbohydrate is not available (as in starvation) or cannot be utilized (as in uncontrolled diabetes) potassium comes out of the cells.

The treatment of potassium intoxication is a matter of urgency. The following measures are used:

1. Glucose and insulin. When glucose enters cells under the influence of insulin, potassium follows. 50 ml of 50 per cent glucose is usually given intravenously. The effect is temporary, because once the glucose has been metabolized, the potassium comes out again. The effect is rapid, however, and buys time for other measures to be instituted.

2. Sodium bicarbonate. In acidotic patients, potassium is displaced from cells by hydrogen ions. Correction of the acidosis by infusion of 500 ml of isotonic (1.26 per cent) sodium bicarbonate induces hydrogen ions to leave the cells, allowing potassium to re-enter.

3. Resonium A. This is a cation exchange resin which releases sodium and hydrogen ions in exchange for potassium ions; the bound potassium ions are then excreted in the faeces. The calcium phase of this resin releases calcium instead of sodium, and is to be preferred in patients whose sodium intake requires careful control. Resonium may be given orally, or by rectal retention enema.

4. If the above measures fail to control the situation, dialysis should be instituted as a matter of urgency. Either haemodialysis or peritoneal dialysis will prove effective, but peritoneal dialysis can usually be set up more rapidly than haemodialysis in an emergency situation.

5. If cardiac arrest is imminent, 20 ml of 10 per cent calcium gluconate should be given intravenously over 2 minutes while preparations are being made for dialysis. Calcium is a physiological antagonist of potassium. If given rapidly in large doses, however, it may itself cause cardiac arrest. For this reason it should be used only in real emergencies.

Disturbances of salt and water balance
(a) Sodium overload. Some patients with renal failure retain

sodium and become overloaded with salt and water. They become oedematous and hypertensive and are liable to develop left ventricular failure and hypertensive encephalopathy. If hypertension is allowed to continue untreated it produces further damage in the already diseased kidneys and accelerates the deterioration of renal function.

Patients who retain sodium are treated with a low salt diet and diuretics. They often require hypotensive drugs in addition. In the presence of renal failure, diuretics in normal doses are often ineffective, but a useful response can usually be obtained with frusemide in doses of 250 to 500 mg. It is important to tailor the sodium content of the diet and the dosage of diuretic to the needs of the individual patient. If this is not done, sodium depletion and hypotension may result, adding a pre-renal element to the renal uraemia already present.

(b) Sodium depletion. In some patients, the kidneys are unable to conserve sodium. These patients usually have a disease (such as chronic pyelonephritis) where the tubules are more severely damaged than the glomeruli. Water is lost in the urine along with salt. The blood pressure falls, and the glomerular filtration rate is reduced, increasing the degree of uraemia.

'Salt wasters' require sodium supplements. The precise amount required must be determined for each patient individually. Sodium depletion is usually accompanied by acidosis, and about half of the sodium supplement is usually given in the form of sodium bicarbonate.

Patients who have difficulty in retaining sodium can become severely uraemic after even a mild gastro-intestinal disturbance, requiring hospital admission and intravenous fluids to restore their electrolyte balance. In spite of this, they often survive for prolonged periods on conservative therapy. This is because hypertension is rarely a problem in these patients, and in the absence of hypertension, the progression of renal disease is often very gradual.

(c) Water intoxication. Patients with renal failure excrete a water load more slowly than individuals with normal kidneys. In spite of this, it is usually both safe and desirable for these patients to have a high fluid intake. The ability to produce a dilute urine is preserved till a late stage in renal failure, and water diuresis promotes the excretion of urea.

84

Eventually a stage is reached where a water load cannot be excreted at all. The urine output becomes considerably less than the fluid intake, and the serum sodium concentration falls, on account of dilution. Cerebral oedema follows, often with drowsiness, confusion and epileptiform convulsions.

The presence of a low serum sodium concentration in a patient who is not clinically dehydrated usually indicates dilution due to water overload. It is a signal to reduce the intake of water.

Metabolic acidosis

During normal metabolism about 60 mEq of 'fixed acid' is produced daily. In chronic renal failure, the ability to excrete hydrogen ions is impaired, and a metabolic acidosis develops. This leads to overbreathing, with a respiratory alkalosis compensating for the metabolic acidosis.

Balance studies have indicated that most patients with chronic renal failure produce about 20 mEq of hydrogen ion more than they can eliminate each day. The serum bicarbonate tends to fall to about 15 mEq per litre and (oddly enough) often remains at about this level, despite continuing accumulation of hydrogen ions in the body. It is thought that buffering of hydrogen ions occurs in bone.

The metabolic acidosis of renal failure is treated by giving oral supplements of sodium bicarbonate.

Treatment of Chronic Renal Failure

The principles of treatment in chronic renal failure are as follows:

1. A high fluid intake should be given.

2. The protein content of the diet should be limited, in order to reduce the amount of nitrogenous waste requiring excretion.

3. Hypertension should be controlled, using salt restriction, diuretics and hypotensive drugs.

4. Abnormalities of electrolyte balance should be detected and corrected. The optimum intake of sodium, bicarbonate and potassium will vary from patient to patient.

5. As soon as it becomes apparent that a patient is progressing towards terminal uraemia, a decision should be made on whether he is a suitable candidate for dialysis or transplantation. If dialysis is decided on — either as a definitive treatment or as a prelude to

a renal transplant — this form of therapy should be started while the patient is still reasonably fit.

Dietary treatment

Sodium, potassium and bicarbonate requirements vary from patient to patient, and must be determined for each individual.

Many of the features of uraemia can be alleviated by reducing the amount of waste material requiring excretion. Carbohydrate and fat are broken down to carbon dioxide and water. The breakdown of protein, however, produces urea and other nitrogenous substances, and also 'fixed acid' which has to be eliminated by the kidneys. Reduction of protein intake reduces the accumulation of nitrogenous waste and hydrogen ions in the body. Figure 18 shows the relationship between the blood urea level and the dietary intake of protein at various glomerular filtration rates.

Patients wih blood urea levels of under 100 mg per cent do not require protein restriction. Patients with blood urea levels of over 150 mg per cent should usually have the dietary protein limited to between 30 and 40 g daily. Provided that a high calorie intake is ensured, most patients with a creatinine clearance of 10 ml per minute or more can be kept in reasonable health with protein restriction of this order. If adequate calories are not supplied, however, body protein will be burned for energy — leading to wasting and emaciation, and increasing the release of nitrogenous waste products.

Patients with creatinine clearances of 5 ml per minute or less are seldom able to tolerate a protein intake of more than 20 g per day without becoming severely uraemic. When the protein content of the diet is as low as this, it is important that as much of the protein as possible be first class — i.e. derived from animal sources. Second class protein (derived from vegetable sources) lacks certain essential amino acids, and cannot be used by the body except as a source of energy. In an 'ordinary' 20 g protein diet, perhaps half the protein is in the form of second class protein such as gluten — the main protein present in wheat bread. The supply of essential amino acids in the diet becomes insufficient to maintain normal muscle bulk and normal plasma protein levels, and the patient becomes extremely emaciated.

It is possible to maintain patients with creatinine clearances as low as 2 ml per minute in reasonable health on 20 g protein, high calorie diets — provided that almost all the protein present in the

86

diet is first class. This is achieved by eliminating vegetable protein from the diet by measures such as the substitution of gluten-free bread for ordinary bread. With artificial diets of this kind it is important to give adequate vitamin supplements.

Once the glomerular filtration rate is less than 5 per cent of normal, the amount of time which can be bought — even with the strictest dietary control in the most co-operative patient — is limited. On average, dietary measures alone can prolong life for about a year. To obtain more prolonged survival in this group of patients, it is necessary to undertake either long-term haemodialysis or renal transplantation.

FAILURE OF TUBULAR FUNCTION

Glomerular disease of any severity is usually associated with impaired function of the renal tubules. Destruction of glomeruli leads to a reduction in the number of nephrons. Hypertrophy of the remaining tubules follows, but this is, as a rule, insufficient to compensate for the reduced number. Each tubule has to operate under the influence of an osmotic diuresis, and as a result concentration, acidification and the reabsorption of filtered ions is interfered with to a greater or lesser extent.

Where the greatest degree of damage occurs in the renal medulla, impairment of renal concentrating power, hydrogen ion excretion, and sodium and potassium reabsorption may be out of proportion to the reduction in glomerular filtration rate.

There are a number of situations in which severe impairment in tubular function may occur before there is any overall loss in renal function. Some of these conditions are acquired, but many of the specific disorders of renal tubular function are congenital.

Single Defects in Tubular Function

1. Renal glycosuria

Here glucose appears in the urine in the presence of a normal blood glucose concentration. There is impaired proximal tubular ability to reabsorb glucose. Renal glycosuria is an inherited disorder. It must be distinguished from diabetes mellitus. Apart from this, it is of little clinical importance.

2. Nephrogenic diabetes insipidus

Diabetes insipidus of pituitary origin can occur at any age. Nephrogenic diabetes insipidus has its onset in early childhood or infancy. There is no response to antidiuretic hormone. It is a rare, inherited condition and appears to be a sex-linked, Mendelian recessive disorder, occurring predominantly in males.

Infants with this condition can become severely dehydrated; many may succumb before they are diagnosed. Those who survive are often mentally deficient. It is thought that brain damage occurs as the result of severe dehydration. Salt depletion (produced by a low salt diet or the administration of diuretics) will lessen the severity of the polyuria. The key point in management is to ensure an adequate fluid intake.

3. Inability to reabsorb phosphate

This condition is sometimes known as vitamin D resistant rickets. There is impaired absorption of calcium from the gastro-intestinal tract, and this is not corrected by physiological amounts of vitamin D. The serum phosphate level is low; despite this the renal clearance of phosphate is abnormally high. Clinical presentation is, as a rule, at about the age of 6 years, with rickets of unusually late onset. Most cases are boys, but female relatives of patients may show a low serum phosphate, in the absence of bone changes. Vitamin D resistant rickets appears to be a sex-linked condition, fully developed in the male, but occurring in a mild, even subclinical form in the female.

Most cases will respond to large doses of vitamin D (e.g. 2 to 5 mg of calciferol daily). It may be necessary to give calcium and phosphate supplements in addition.

Following vitamin D therapy, phosphate reabsorption in the renal tubules often improves. It is thought that the high phosphate excretion in this condition may be the result of hyperparathyroidism secondary to impaired calcium absorption in the gut.

4. Inability to reabsorb calcium

This condition is also known as idiopathic hypercalciuria. It is discussed in Chapter 9, as a cause of renal calculi.

5. Inability to reabsorb cystine, and other amino acids

In this congenital condition, there is a specific defect in the tubular reabsorptive mechanism shared by cystine, lysine, arginine and ornithine. Abnormal amounts of these amino acids appear in the urine. Cystine is the most insoluble of these substances, and the importance of the condition lies in the formation of cystine calculi. Cystinuria is discussed in Chapter 9.

Multiple Defects of Tubular Function

Fanconi syndrome

Here there is defective reabsorption of glucose, phosphate and amino acids. In addition, there is proteinuria, and an impaired ability to concentrate the urine or to excrete hydrogen ion. The blood urea rises gradually, as glomerular function becomes increasingly impaired.

Microdissection of renal tubules shows a rather striking abnormality. The proximal tubule is abnormally short, and is connected to the glomerulus by a long thin 'neck'.

The Fanconi syndrome may occur in children or in adults. Childhood cases occur in association with *cystinosis* – the production of abnormally large amounts of cystine, associated with cystine deposition at many sites in the body. Inheritance of cystinosis is as a Mendelian recessive trait.

Adult cases also appear to be familial, but are not associated with cystinosis.

Renal tubular acidosis

This condition may be congenital or acquired. The kidneys are unable to produce a hydrogen ion gradient between the tubular fluid and the plasma, and as a result an acid urine cannot be excreted. There is also inability to concentrate the urine.

Inability to excrete hydrogen ions produces a metabolic acidosis. Less calcium than normal is bound to protein and this increases the filtration of calcium at the glomeruli. The tubular fluid is abnormally alkaline, and this leads to the precipitation of calcium salts in the renal substance (nephrocalcinosis) and to the formation of calcium stones in the urinary tract.

Treatment of renal tubular acidosis is with bicarbonate supplements.

Renal Failure and Potassium Depletion

Renal disease may cause potassium depletion.

Potassium depletion arising from extra-renal mechanisms may

cause renal lesions. Causes of potassium depletion are shown in Table 3.

Potassium depletion produces specific lesions in the renal tubular cells. These consist of multiple, well-demarcated vacuoles situated within the cytoplasm. If potassium depletion is severe and prolonged 'interstitial nephritis' occurs, inflammatory cells infiltrate the renal interstitium, and fibrosis of the parenchyma ensues. It is thought by some authorities that pyelonephritis occurs as a complication of potassium depletion more often than would be expected on the basis of chance.

Table 3 Causes of potassium depletion

Renal Causes
1. Diuretic phase of acute tubular necrosis.
2. Diuretic response to the relief of urinary tract obstruction.
3. Implantation of ureter in large bowel.
4. Renal tubular acidosis.
5. Renal artery stenosis (due to secondary aldosteronism; see Chapter 7).
6. Chronic renal failure due to any cause; especially when urine volume is high.

Extra-renal Causes
1. Prolonged vomiting (as in pyloric stenosis) or prolonged gastric suction.
2. Prolonged diarrhoea – e.g. malabsorption syndrome, misuse of purgatives.
3. Any condition in which there is a systemic alkalosis. (Potassium is excreted in place of hydrogen ion in the reabsorption of sodium.)
4. Intestinal and biliary fistulae.
5. Diuretic administration.
6. Primary aldosteronism (Conn's syndrome).
7. Secondary aldosteronism (e.g. cardiac failure, nephrotic syndrome, ascites).
8. Uncontrolled diabetes mellitus.

Potassium depletion leads to the development of muscular weakness; in the very severe case paralysis and death from respiratory failure may occur. Patients are apathetic, anorexic and confused. Digitalis toxicity is intensified. If a patient on digitalis therapy becomes potassium-depleted, a variety of arrhythmias (including ventricular fibrillation) may occur.

Thirst and polyuria are prominent symptoms. The ability to produce a concentrated urine is lost, and hypotonic urine may be produced in the presence of an osmotically concentrated plasma. This situation is not reversed by the administration of antidiuretic hormone. The blood urea level rises – partly as the result of impaired renal blood flow resulting from dehydration, and partly as the result of increased back-diffusion of urea into the blood from the proximal tubule.

In its early stages renal failure due to potassium depletion can be reversed by rehydration and the correction of the potassium deficit. Once interstitial inflammation and fibrosis have occurred, however, only partial reversal of the situation can be expected.

Hypercalcaemia as a Cause of Renal Failure

An excess of calcium – whether it be in the blood or in the tubular fluid – can lead to marked impairment in renal function. Hypercalcaemia causes degenerative changes in renal tubular cells – particularly in the collecting ducts and distal tubules. These early changes are associated with loss of concentrating ability by the kidney; polyuria and polydipsia are common.

If a high serum calcium persists, the damaged tubular cells become necrotic, slough and become calcified. Calcified casts obstruct the collecting ducts. As a result of the obstruction produced by these casts, renal failure develops. In its early stages, the renal failure can be reversed by lowering the serum calcium level. If hypercalcaemia is allowed to persist, however, calcium is deposited in the renal substance itself. This deposition is termed *nephrocalcinosis* (Chap. 9). The obstructed tubules undergo atrophy throughout their length, and the associated glomeruli become replaced by fibrous tissue. Once these changes have occurred, the recovery which follows correction of the serum calcium level is far from complete.

If the serum calcium level is *very* high (15–20 mg per cent) 'hypercalcaemic crisis' may ensue, affecting many systems in the body. There is anorexia, vomiting, extreme lethargy and a stuporose mental state which may progress to coma. Cardiac arrest may occur. If renal function remains reasonably good, the serum calcium level may be lowered by the intravenous infusion of sodium versenate – the sodium salt of ethylene tetra-amino acetic acid (EDTA). If renal function is impaired, intravenous sodium phosphate can be used. These measures are only temporarily effective and definitive treatment consists in correcting the cause of hypercalcaemia.

The causes of hypercalcaemia and hypercalciuria are discussed in Chapter 9.

FURTHER READING

Merrill, J. P. (1963). Acute renal failure. In *Diseases of the Kidney.* Ed. Strauss, M. B. & Welt, L. G. London: Churchill.

Milne, M. D. (1963). Renal tubular dysfunction. *Ibid.*

Rosenheim, M. L. & Ross, E. J. Chronic renal failure. *Ibid.*

Schreiner, G. E. (1967). Acute renal failure. In *Renal Disease,* 2nd ed. Ed. Black, D. A. K. Oxford: Blackwell.

Chapter 5

DIALYSIS AND TRANSPLANTATION

In some cases renal failure can be managed conservatively. The intake of fluids, salts and nitrogen-containing foods can be adjusted to quantities which the damaged kidneys are able to handle without the production of severe metabolic imbalance.

Careful conservative treatment can tide a patient with mild acute renal failure over his period of oliguria, allowing him to survive until the kidneys recover. Infected or traumatized cases tend to be hypercatabolic, however, and when the blood urea level is rising by 100 mg per cent per day, conservative methods of therapy are doomed to failure.

In chronic renal failure a co-operative patient, carefully managed, can survive for months or even years on conservative treatment with a glomerular filtration rate as low as 3 ml per minute, but sooner or later all useful renal function is lost. The alternatives then are death, dialysis or transplantation.

DIALYSIS

The principles of dialysis are simple. Given a semi-permeable membrane with the patient's blood on one side and a solution of known composition on the other, substances to which the membrane is permeable will move from where their concentration is high to where their concentration is low. If the blood urea level is high, and urea is absent from the dialysis solution, urea will pass from the blood to the solution. If the blood sodium level is low, and the sodium concentration in the dialysis solution is in the normal range, sodium will pass from the solution into the blood. By using a dialysis solution which contains the important electrolytes in concentrations which are normal for healthy individuals, the concentration of these electrolytes can be corrected in the blood of the patient with renal failure. Since waste products like urea, uric acid and creatinine are absent from the

93

dialysis solution, dialysis will remove these substances from the patient's blood.

Dialysis can be carried out either within the patient's body, using the peritoneum as the dialysis membrane, or outside the patient's body, using an artificial kidney machine and a membrane such as cellophane.

Peritoneal Dialysis

Here a cannula is introduced into the peritoneal cavity and attached to a three-way tap. Sterile dialysis fluid is run into the peritoneum, and allowed to equilibrate with blood for about 20 minutes. The fluid is then drained, and the cycle is repeated by running in fresh fluid.

In addition to correcting the concentrations of electrolytes and removing waste products, dialysis can be used to remove fluid from overhydrated patients. In peritoneal dialysis, this is done by adding glucose to the dialysis fluid until it is hypertonic with respect to plasma. Water moves across membranes more rapidly than glucose, and the hypertonic dialysis fluids act osmotically to suck fluid out of the patient. If the patient is not overhydrated, isotonic fluid can be used.

Peritoneal dialysis has the advantage of requiring little in the way of specialized equipment. It has the disadvantage of being uncomfortable for the patient; it also carries a definite risk of peritonitis. Between 20 and 40 g of protein are lost from the body during a 24-hour peritoneal dialysis, and this protein must be replaced by the intravenous infusion of 2 or more pints of plasma or blood during the procedure. Water-soluble vitamins are also lost during dialysis, and supplements of these should be given. Using peritoneal dialysis in the average adult it takes about 24 hours to halve the blood urea level. If the patient is hyper-catabolic, producing urea at a rapid rate, peritoneal dialysis may not succeed in doing more than holding the biochemistry steady. In such patients haemodialysis using an artificial kidney machine is necessary.

In chronic renal failure, peritoneal dialysis may be used to keep the patient alive while the full situation is assessed. It is not an acceptable method of achieving long-term survival, however. Adhesions make the procedure increasingly less effective as time goes on, and peritonitis becomes less of a risk and more of a certainty. Quite apart from the technical considerations, although most patients can tolerate the discomfort of 3 or 4 treatments, few can put up with 6 months of twice weekly peritoneal dialysis without becoming demoralized. The hours spent in hospital preclude a normal home and working life, and the patient is never free from discomfort for more than a day or two at a time.

Haemodialysis

Here dialysis takes place outside the body, and some form or other of kidney machine is used. A kidney machine consists simply of a semi-permeable membrane with blood on one side and dialysis fluid on the other. Various permutations and combinations have been tried with a view to improving performance, but two basic types of artificial kidney exist, both of which employ either cellophane or the closely related substance cuprophane as the dialysis membrane.

The Kolff artificial kidney consists of a coil, or rather (to increase surface area and reduce resistance to flow) of two coils arranged in parallel. Blood is pumped through the inside of the coil, and dialysis fluid is pumped around the outside (Fig. 19).

The Kiil artificial kidney is sometimes known as the 'sandwich machine'. Two cellophane sheets clamped round their edges form an envelope; to increase surface area two or more envelopes of this kind are arranged in parallel (Fig. 20).

All parts of the machine with which the blood comes in contact are sterile. The dialysis side of the membrane need not be sterile, as bacteria are too large to pass through the membrane. Bacterial toxins can cross, however, and there is some doubt about whether the membrane is completely impermeable at all times to the virus of infectious hepatitis. For these reasons, attempts are made to render the entire machine as free from organisms as possible.

As with peritoneal dialysis, substances pass from where their concentration is high to where it is low. Fluid can be removed from the body by making the dialysis fluid hypertonic, as with peritoneal dialysis, but a technique known as ultrafiltration is also used. By pumping the blood through under high pressure and sucking the dialysis fluid through under negative pressure, the hydrostatic pressure on the blood side of the membrane can be made 200 mm Hg or more greater than that on the dialysis fluid

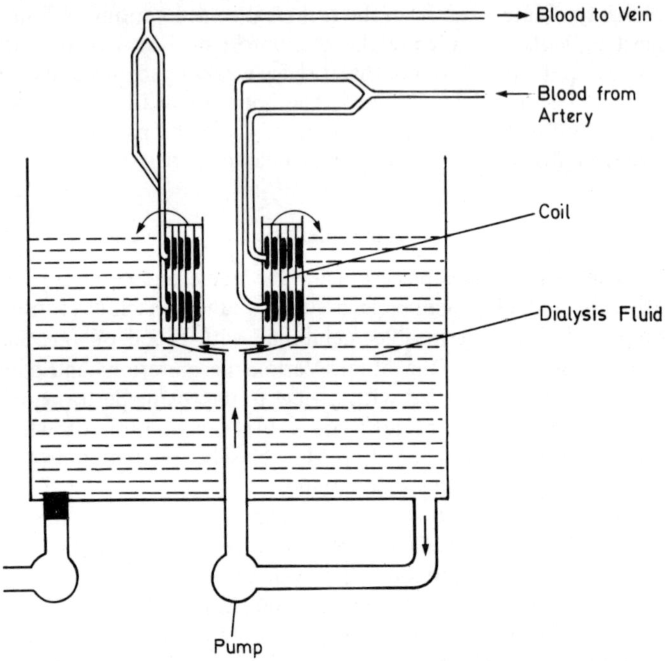

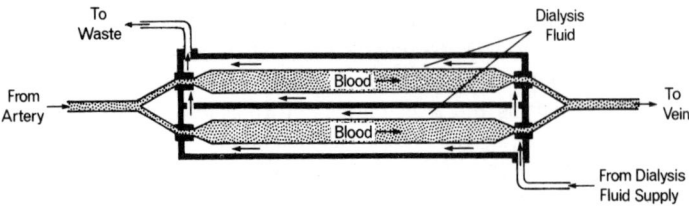

Fig. 19. Diagram of the twin coil (Kolff) artificial kidney machine.

side. This leads to salt and water being forced hydrostatically out of the blood into the dialysis fluid.

The artificial kidney was invented over 20 years ago, and has been in use for the treatment of acute renal failure since the Second World War. Its successful use in chronic renal failure, however, goes back only about 10 years. This is because of the

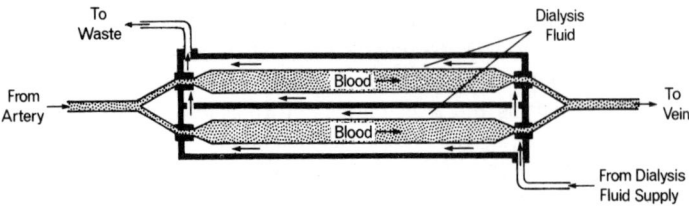

Fig. 20. Diagram of the Kiil dialyser (for explanation see text).

problem of getting blood out of the patient and back in again at a rate of between 100 and 200 ml per minute. Flow rates of this kind can be achieved by cannulating an artery and a large vein. Such cannulae can be kept open for days or weeks by the injection of heparin, but eventually they clot and become infected. In 1960 Scribner described a shunt constructed of teflon and siliconized rubber which took blood from an artery and returned it to a vein (Fig. 21). The flow in such shunts is rapid enough to minimize the risk of clotting. When the patient is dialysed, the shunt is taken apart; at the end of dialysis, it is reconstituted.

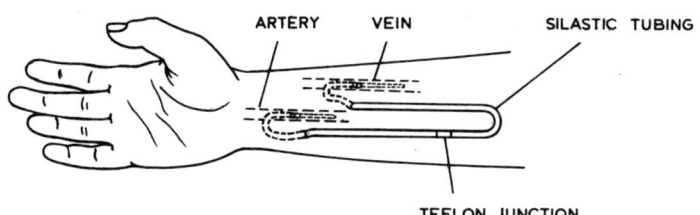

Fig. 21. The Scribner-Quinton arteriovenous shunt.

More recently, use has been made of an arteriovenous fistula, constructed by anastomosing an artery directly to a vein. After a few weeks of rapid high pressure flow, the vein dilates. 'Venepuncture' with very large needles becomes easy, and gives access to rapidly flowing blood under arterial pressure.

To prevent clotting in the machine, the blood is anticoagulated with heparin.

Patients with chronic renal failure are dialysed at least twice a week, for 10 to 14 hours on each occasion. The blood urea levels at the start of dialysis are seldom above 160 mg per cent; by the end of dialysis urea levels of 60 mg per cent or less are usual.

Although it is easy to obtain reasonable biochemical control in dialysis patients, the artificial kidney does not manufacture erythropoietin, and anaemia is universal, the haemoglobin level being between 40 and 55 per cent as a rule. Attempts to maintain higher levels by repeated transfusions have been abandoned, partly because of transfusion reactions, and partly because of the serious risk of hepatitis involved with multiple transfusions. Despite the anaemia most patients with chronic renal failure who are on regular dialysis therapy can be rehabilitated and returned to full-time employment.

Dialysis techniques are becoming simpler, cheaper and more automated. Hundreds of patients are now dialysed in their own homes.

TRANSPLANTATION

The idea of transplantation is not new. St Damien carried out leg transplantation many centuries ago, but that was either a myth or a miracle. Branca carried out nasal transplantation in the 15th century; when the donors died, however, the grafts fell off the faces of the recipients. This masterpiece of medieval surgery can be regarded as truly legendary. We are on more factual ground in the 18th century. John Hunter transplanted the testis of a cock in 1771; he noted, however, that the disposition of the recipient hen was not altered.

In the 19th century, skin transplantation in human subjects was introduced. Skin autografts (i.e. transfer of skin from one site to another in the same patient) were found to be successful; skin homografts (the grafting of skin from another individual of the same species) took temporarily, and were then rejected. In 1927, however, it was found that skin homografts between identical twins would take permanently. These observations led on to the concept of genetically based tissue tolerance.

In 1952, Murray reported 6 cases of renal transplantation in man; the donors were cadavers unrelated to the recipients. All the grafts failed, but 3 functioned for over a month. Although these results were not clinically useful, they showed that renal transplantation was technically feasible, and in 1956 Murray and Merrill carried out renal transplantation between identical twins, with excellent graft function, prolonged survival and restoration of normal health. Only one person in every 90 is an identical twin, however, and it was not possible to apply the technique of transplantation with success to the general problem of chronic renal failure until a method had been found to deal with the problem of graft rejection.

Initial attempts at modifying the rejection process were by subjecting the recipients to massive doses of body irradiation. This technique was reasonably effective in suppressing the immune response to foreign tissue; a few patients treated in this way 10 years ago are still alive today. Unfortunately, it also

98

resulted in almost complete abolition of all resistance to infection, and the morbidity and mortality of this method of immuno-suppression soon led to its being abandoned.

Now the standard way of combating rejection is by combined therapy with azothiaprine (Imuran) and prednisone. Lymphocytes are of great importance in the rejection phenomenon, and these drugs are sometimes supplemented by antilymphocytic globulin, produced by immunizing animals (usually horses) against human lymphocytes.

The kidney graft is placed in one or other iliac fossa. The renal vessels are anastomosed to the iliac vessels, and the donor ureter is introduced into the patient's bladder (Fig. 22).

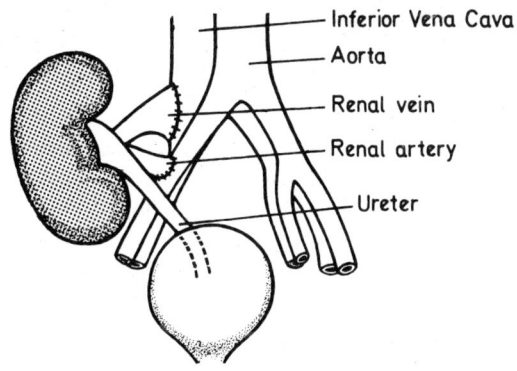

Fig. 22. Renal transplantation in the right iliac fossa.

One problem is that the transplanted kidney is without a blood supply for a variable period of time. This leads to a greater or lesser degree of tubular necrosis. Transplants from living related donors can be carried out electively, and the time that the kidney is ischaemic can be kept to an hour or less. When cadavers are used as a source of kidneys for transplantation, however, there may be considerable delay in getting the kidney to the patient and vice versa. Provided the graft is removed from a cavader within an hour of death and chilled to $4^{\circ}C$, it can be kept for about 10 hours in its chilled state and still give excellent function – eventually. With long ischaemia times, however, a fairly prolonged period of tubular necrosis can be expected, and many patients receiving cadaver grafts require post-operative dialysis for between 1 and 4 weeks.

It is thought that the antigens which are important in rejection are present in white blood cells as well as in the kidneys, and about 13 important human leucocyte antigens have now been recognized. By carrying out white cell typing pre-operatively, it is possible to avoid the transplantation of grossly incompatible kidneys; but the extent to which tissue typing has improved the prognosis in transplantation has not yet been fully worked out.

There is less genetic incompatibility between living related donors and recipients than there is between unrelated cadavers and recipients, and with living donors the operation can be elective. Recent results indicate that over 80 per cent of grafts from living relatives will be functioning at the end of 1 year. With cadaver donors the results are less good. Five years ago only 20 per cent of cadaver grafts survived 1 year; now the figure is over 45 per cent 1-year survival for such grafts. A graft which is functioning well at the end of 1 year stands an odds-on chance of being functional at the end of 5.

In spite of the fact that living donor results are considerably better than results with cadaver transplants, most transplant surgeons are unwilling to subject healthy subjects to an operation with an appreciable morbidity which is not for their benefit. For this reason most kidney transplants (in Britain, at any rate) utilize cadaver kidneys.

Comparison of Dialysis and Transplantation

The best treatment for chronic renal failure is a successful renal transplant, but not all transplants are successful. Transplanted patients tend to be Cushingoid from steroid therapy, and they are liable to infection, as their immunity has been tampered with. On the other hand, they do not have to spend 28 hours a week being dialysed, they are not anaemic, and their quality of life is much better than that of the average dialysis patient.

In the past, there were arguments about the relative merits of dialysis and transplantation, but it now seems that the premises of these arguments were mistaken. With about 50 per million of the population under the age of 55 developing irreversible renal failure annually, the only way in which the problem can be tackled is by dialysis *and* transplantation. Patients are dialysed till they are fit for operation, and are then transplanted. If the graft fails, they are returned to dialysis – perhaps to await a second transplant.

FURTHER READING

Calne, R. Y. (1967). *Renal Transplantation,* 2nd ed. London: Arnold.
Nolan, B. (1967). Transplantation of the kidney. In *Renal Disease,* 2nd ed. Ed. Black, D. A. K. Oxford: Blackwell.
Scribner, B. H. (1967). Dialysis. *Ibid.*

Chapter 6

THE KIDNEYS AND HYPERTENSION

PHYSIOLOGICAL CONSIDERATIONS

Some renal diseases cause hypertension, and hypertension – especially when severe – can produce renal damage. In many instances it is impossible to be certain whether hypertension is secondary to renal disease or vice versa.

Experimental Renal Hypertension

In 1827, Bright and Bostock showed that proteinuric patients tended to become hypertensive, and to have small, granular kidneys on autopsy. A relationship between the kidneys and the blood pressure was shown more directly in 1898, when Tigerstedt and Bergman produced high blood pressure in animals by the injection of extracts of renal tissue. In 1934, Goldblatt produced hypertension in dogs and rats by a variety of techniques involving the occlusion of a renal artery. In dogs, to produce hypertension it was necessary to obstruct one renal artery partially and also to remove the opposite kidney. In the rat, a high blood pressure could be produced by the partial obstruction of one renal artery alone, leaving the contralateral kidney intact.

In the rat, Goldblatt found that if the occluded kidney was either removed or had its blood supply restored, the blood pressure would return to normal – provided that the correction was carried out early enough. If hypertension had been allowed to persist, however, these measures did not restore the blood pressure to normal, because persistent high blood pressure produced irreversible damage in the non-obstructed kidney. It was later found that even persistent hypertension could be relieved in this situation by removal of the non-occluded kidney, coupled by restoration of a normal blood supply to the occluded kidney. The explanation of this apparent paradox is that although the non-occluded kidney is irreversibly damaged by the hypertension, the partial obstruction of the renal artery on the occluded side protects this kidney from the high systemic pressure.

Soon after the publication of Goldblatt's experiments, a man was cured of high blood pressure by the removal of a unilateral pyelonephritic kidney. This stimulated a great deal of work on renal hypertension in man, but the early results were rather baffling, and the effects of many of the nephrectomies carried out for the relief of hypertension were disappointing. We still understand only part of the story, but it now appears that primary renal hypertension is initiated through the action of an enzyme known as renin which is produced at the juxtaglomerular apparatus of the kidneys.

The Role of Renin in the Production of Hypertension

Renin is a protein with a molecular weight of about 45,000, produced by the juxtaglomerular apparatus. This structure (Fig. 23) is situated in the angle between the afferent and efferent

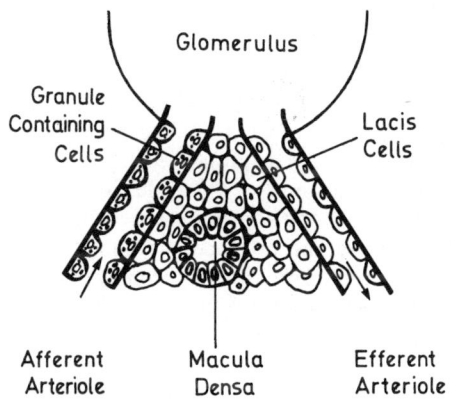

Fig. 23. The juxtaglomerular apparatus (for explanation see text).

arterioles of the glomerulus, in close relationship to a segment of the distal tubule known as the macula densa. The area bounded by the two arterioles and the macula densa contains clear cells known as lacis cells. The walls of the afferent arteriole in the neighbourhood of the juxtaglomerular apparatus contain secretory granules, and it is thought that these granules consist of

103

renin. Renin is an enzyme and not a hormone. It acts on angiotensinogen (a substance produced in the liver) to give angiotensin I. Angiotensin I is a polypeptide of 10 amino acids which is converted in the plasma to a substance known as angiotensin II, consisting of 8 amino acids. Angiotensin II is the most powerful pressor substance known, and it is the agent responsible for the rise in blood pressure which follows the release of renin. It acts to raise the blood pressure in two ways. Firstly, it has a direct constrictor effect on blood vessels; secondly, it stimulates the release of aldosterone from the adrenal cortex. Aldosterone promotes sodium retention, which increases the volume of extracellular fluid in the body, and raises the blood pressure as a result.

The stimulus to the release of renin from the juxtaglomerular apparatus appears to be a fall in hydrostatic pressure at the afferent arteriole. A fall in pressure at this site may be due to:

1. A low blood pressure in the aorta.
2. Narrowing of the renal artery.
3. Narrowing of the renal arterioles themselves – as may occur in a wide range of parenchymal diseases of the kidney.

A low plasma sodium concentration may also act as a stimulus for renin release.

The renin/angiotensin system and aldosterone prodction are kept in equilibrium by a negative feed-back mechanism mediated partly through the arterial pressure and partly through the sodium content of the body. When aldosterone production is abnormally low (as in Addison's disease) renin production is increased. When aldosterone production is increased (as in Conn's syndrome) plasma renin levels are abnormally low. In salt-wasting renal disease, however, when the kidneys do not respond to aldosterone, the plasma levels of renin and aldosterone are both increased.

It is generally agreed that renin is the major cause of renal hypertension. What *maintains* it, however, is a mystery, because in severe and long-standing renal hypertension plasma renin levels are often normal. One theory is that the baroreceptors, which signal to the brain whether or not the blood pressure is normal, become 'reset' at a higher level if hypertension has been present for some time, and a high blood pressure is then regarded by the body as 'normal'. An alternative explanation, for which there is some experimental evidence, is that some hypertensive patients become abnormally sensitive to the pressor effects of angiotensin II, and normal plasma renin levels are then sufficient to maintain hypertension. This is particularly likely to arise if the sodium content of the body is abnormally high.

The role of renin in the control of blood pressure is summarized in Table 4.

Table 4 Renin in the control of blood pressure

1. *Low blood pressure* (in afferent arteriole)   Release of RENIN from
        or   ⟶   juxtaglomerular
   Low plasma volume   apparatus

2. *Angiotensinogen* (an alpha 2 globulin also known as 'renin substrate')

                  ↓   RENIN

   Angiotensin 1 (decapeptide)

                  ↓

   Angiotensin 2 (active agent, octapeptide)

3. *Angiotensin 2*
   - (a) stimulates aldosterone secretion by the adrenal cortex
   - (b) increases blood pressure by direct action on vessels
   - (c) increases sympathetic tone by acting on central nervous system

4. *Aldosterone*
   promotes sodium reabsorption in the distal tubule

5. *Sodium retention*
   - (a) expands plasma volume and increases blood pressure
   - (b) by expanding plasma volume, acts to *reduce* renin secretion

6. *In healthy subjects*
   restoration of a normal blood pressure –
   improves perfusion through the afferent arterioles and *decreases* renin production

7. *In some disease states* (e.g. malignant hypertension)
   a rise in blood pressure –
   may *increase* renin production by causing arteriolar damage

Causes of Hypertension

Essential hypertension

A precipitating cause cannot be found in most patients with hypertension; in this situation the hypertension is called *essential.*

Renal hypertension

Only 15 per cent of cases of hypertension are due to renal disease. Almost any parenchymal disorder of the kidneys, bilateral or unilateral, can cause hypertension. The detection of cases due to unilateral renal disease is important, because removal of the diseased kidney may cure the hypertension. Renal artery stenosis is an example of a cause of hypertension which may be cured by surgery.

Coarctation of the aorta
In this condition a segment of the aorta — usually in the thorax, below the arch — is narrowed, and blood reaches the lower half of the body by devious anastomotic channels. The pressure in the afferent arterioles is reduced and hypertension occurs. This hypertension is confined to those parts which are supplied from the aorta proximal to the stenosis.

Polycythaemia
Hypertension is usually a feature of polycythaemia vera.

Endocrine causes
Certain rare endocrine causes of hypertension assume a degree of importance out of proportion to their frequency because the hypertension they cause can often be cured by surgery.

Adrenal cortical diseases
In *Cushing's syndrome* hypertension is due to the over-production of gluco-corticoids.

In *Conn's syndrome* there is hypertrophy of the glomerulosa cells of the adrenal cortex and overproduction of the mineralo-corticoid, aldosterone.

The *adrenogenital syndrome* is characterized by over-production of sex hormones by the adrenals. These hormones have many effects, but the production of serious hypertension is not one of them. In a few cases of the adrenogenital syndrome, however, there is also overproduction of aldosterone.

Adrenal medullary diseases
Phaeochromocytoma is a tumour of the adrenal medulla or sympathetic ganglia. It causes hypertension by overproduction of adrenaline and noradrenaline.

Investigation of Hypertension

The more important investigations are listed in Table 5, and most of these should be carried out in hypertensive patients

106

Table 5 The investigation of hypertension

A *Assessment of the Severity of Hypertension*

The presence of any of the following is an indication for treatment in hypertension:
1. Symptoms attributable to hypertension.
2. Serious elevation of the diastolic blood pressure (e.g. over 120 mm Hg).
3. Cardiac failure attributable to hypertension.
4. Clinical or radiological evidence of left ventricular enlargement.
5. Fundal changes indicating damage to small blood vessels.
6. ECG evidence of left ventricular hypertrophy or strain.
7. Biochemical evidence of impaired renal function.

B *Investigation of the Cause of Hypertension*

Routine investigations (usually performed on an outpatient basis).
1. *Detailed Medical History*
   Particular attention is given to:
   (i) urinary symptoms (these may suggest renal disease or aldosteronism).
   (ii) paroxysmal symptoms (these occur in 50 per cent of patients with phaeochromocytoma).
2. *Physical Examination*
   Particular attention is given to:
   (i) auscultation of the abdomen (a bruit might suggest renal artery stenosis).
   (ii) palpation of the kidneys (gross bilateral enlargement suggests polycystic disease).
   (iii) palpation of the femoral pulses (weak or delayed femoral pulses suggest coarctation of the aorta).
3. *Urine Analysis*
   (i) Test for protein (proteinuria is usually present in diffuse renal disease).
   (ii) Test for sugar (the incidence of hypertension is increased in diabetes, particularly if there is nephropathy).
   (iii) Microscopical examination (abnormalities are common in diffuse renal disease and in urinary tract infection).
   (iv) Bacteriological examination (midstream urine specimens × 3).
4. *Estimation of Plasma Urea and Electrolytes*
   (i) Elevation of the blood urea suggests renal damage.
   (ii) A low plasma K (under 3.6 mEq/l) suggests aldosteronism, unless the patient is on diuretic therapy. (Prolonged tourniquet application during venipuncture must be avoided; this produces falsely high K values.)
   (iii) An elevated bicarbonate level with a low K, is also in favour of aldosteronism.
5. *Full Blood Count and E.S.R.*
   (i) Incidence of hypertension is increased in polycythaemia.
   (ii) Connective tissue disorders (lupus, polyarteritis) are associated with changes in white cell count and ESR.
6. *Creatinine Clearance Determination*
   To assess overall renal function.

Table 5 (continued)

7. *Urinary Excretion of Vanilyl Mandelic Acid (VMA)*
   VMA excretion of over 8 mg/day suggests phaeschromocytoma.
   (The same 24-hour urine collection can be used for VMA
   estimation and creatinine clearance.)

8. *Intravenous Pyelography*
   May reveal chronic pyelonephritis, renal vascular disease, contracted kidneys, polycystic disease etc.

9. *Isotope Renography*
   In conjunction with the intravenous pyelogram, this gives a good
   qualitative assessment of the separate function of the two
   kidneys.

10. *Special Investigations*
    (These requrie hospital admission, but are only required in a very
    small minority of hypertensive patients.)
    (i) *Aortography.* To confirm suspected coarctation of the aorta.
    (ii) *Renal Aortography.* To confirm suspected renal vascular
    disease in young patients.
    (iii) *Percutaneous Renal Biopsy.* To establish the diagnosis in
    diffuse renal disease.
    (iv) *Retroperitoneal Air Insufflation.* In cases of suspected
    adrenal tumour.
    (v) *Divided Renal Function Tests.* Used where removal of one
    kidney is contemplated.

under the age of 50, unless the cause of hypertension is obvious.

In patients over the age of 50, investigations of a specialized
nature are less clearly indicated, because essential hypertension is
overwhelmingly more common than all other causes of hypertension together, and even renal hypertension often responds
better to hypotensive drugs than to surgery in this age group.
There is, however, nothing magical about the age of 50, and the
entire clinical picture must be taken into account when deciding
just how far to press investigations in a particular patient with
hypertension.

For accounts of essential hypertension, phaeochromocytoma,
Cushing's syndrome, coarctation of the aorta and the adrenogenital syndrome, the reader is referred to general medical texts.
Renal artery stenosis and *Conn's syndrome* involve renal
mechanisms and are therefore discussed in the present chapter.

Renal Artery Stenosis

The renal artery may be occluded either by atheroma or by
fibromuscular hyperplasia. If its calibre is reduced by 70 per cent
or more renal ischaemia occurs and hypertension follows. Only
half the patients with hypertension due to renal artery stenosis

have raised plasma renin levels. In the others, although the hypertension was presumably caused by increased renin production, high levels are not required to sustain it.

In renal artery stenosis a systolic bruit may be heard over the affected kidney. In intravenous pyelograms the partially occluded and ischaemic kidney is usually slightly smaller than the opposite, non-occluded one, and excretes the contrast medium more slowly. It often appears more radio-opaque than the normal kidney. This is because the low arteriolar pressure in the stenotic kidney reduces glomerular filtration more than it reduces tubular function and a greater percentage than normal of the glomerular filtrate is reabsorbed. As a result, the contrast medium is more concentrated. Renography is also a useful investigation in cases of suspected renal artery stenosis.

Treatment. If operation is contemplated arteriography is essential, not only to confirm the diagnosis, but also to delineate the site and extent of the obstruction. Divided renal function tests, which involve ureteric catheterization, are sometimes used.

The operation of choice in younger patients is relief of the arterial obstruction without nephrectomy, although nephrectomy is technically simpler. If the hypertension is severe, there may be doubt about the integrity of the 'normal' kidney, especially in older patients in whom essential hypertension may be associated with an atheromatous plaque at the origin of the renal artery. Rather than subject older patients to tedious, and at times dangerous, investigations and operation, it may be simpler to treat the hypertension medically.

Some years ago, when surgery was carried out in almost all cases of renal artery stenosis, the cure rate was about 25 per cent. Now that patients are more carefully selected the cure rate following operation is about 50 per cent. This change in policy has greatly reduced the morbidity from unsuccessful operation and from over-enthusiastic investigation in patients unlikely to benefit from surgery.

Primary Aldosteronism (Conn's Syndrome)

This condition is given more space here than its incidence merits, partly because it can usually be cured by surgical treatment, and partly because of its physiological importance. The glomerulosa cells of the adrenal cortex produce aldosterone. Hyperplasia or an adenoma of these cells causes excessive production of the hormone. Aldosterone promotes sodium reabsorption in exchange for potassium ions in the distal convoluted tubule.

Despite the salt-retaining properties of aldosterone, oedema is rare in Conn's syndrome, and most cases present with hypertension and a low serum potassium. The plasma renin level is low. There are few conditions other than primary aldosteronism in which a low renin and a high aldosterone level coexist.

Secondary aldosteronism complicates many cases of cardiac failure, ascites, the nephrotic syndrome and essential hypertension. It tends to be associated with *high* renin levels.

Effects on the Kidneys of Hypertension

Hypertension produces changes in all arterioles and the severity of these changes is roughly correlated with the severity of the hypertension. Severe changes in the blood vessels of the retina, which can be directly visualized through an ophthalmoscope, tend to be accompanied by equally severe changes in renal vessels.

Mild hypertension produces a moderate thickening of the whole wall of the smaller arterioles, which may persist unchanged for years. In some cases, however, the arterioles narrow sufficiently to produce small wedge-shaped areas of ischaemic degeneration in the kidneys. These ischaemic areas may liberate enough renin to cause a marked increase in the severity of the hypertension. A patient who for years has had a moderately elevated blood pressure with good overall renal function may suddenly develop malignant hypertension, with retinal haemorrhages, retinal exudates, papilloedema and rapidly declining renal function.

Malignant hypertension is associated with gross retinal changes and with a rapid decline in renal function. At first there is marked thickening of the intima of the larger arteries, which are narrowed to a greater or lesser degree. This leads to the release of renin from ischaemic afferent arterioles, and thyblood pressure rises still further. Focal necrosis then occurs in the afferent arterioles, and as the necrosed areas contain fibrin the change is called 'fibrinoid necrosis'. If the blood pressure is allowed to remain elevated, these localized changes became widespread, and almost

110

all renal cells can die very rapidly. In malignant hypertension with falling renal function, lowering the blood pressure is a matter of urgency.

Malignant hypertension can be diagnosed more accurately from the state of the optic fundi than from the height of the diastolic blood pressure, because the rate at which hypertension develops is as important as the height of the blood pressure.

Treatment of Renal Hypertension

The medical treatment of renal hypertension does not differ in principle from that for essential hypertension, but control is required more urgently. The pharmacology of hypotensive drugs, and their relative advantages and disadvantages are discussed adequately in most general medical textbooks.

In essential hypertension, lowering of the blood pressure over a period of several days is usually acceptable. In renal hypertension, however, rapid lowering of the blood pressure may be essential. The following three drugs have the advantage of being rapid in their action. All three have serious disadvantages in long-term use, but are reasonably safe if given for a limited period.

Reserpine can cause severe depression, and may lead to suicide if used for long periods. It will, however, often bring malignant hypertension under rapid control − without producing severe hypotension. 1 mg is given intramuscularly at hourly intervals until the blood pressure comes under control. If two or three 1-mg injections are given with little effect, the dose is increased.

Hydrallizine can produce a collagen disease similar to SLE when given in high dosage for a prolonged period of time. The occasional use of the drug in an emergency, however, does not carry this risk. The dose is 10 mg to 20 mg given intramuscularly or intravenously.

Diazoxide is chemically similar to the thiazide diuretics, but has no diuretic action. It raises the blood sugar level, and when used repeatedly it can produce diabetes. This serious disadvantage precludes its long-term use as a hypotensive agent. It is, however, an invaluable drug in desperate situations where hypertension has produced severe left ventricular failure or convulsions. A single intravenous dose of 300 mg will reduce the blood pressure to normal or near-normal levels within 2 or 3 minutes. The effect lasts between 6 and 24 hours. During this period more

111

conventional hypotensive agents are given to keep the blood pressure under control once the effect of diazoxide has worn off.

FURTHER READING

Lee, M. R. (1969). *Renin and Hypertension.* London: Lloyd-Luke.
Peart, W. S. (1967). Hypertension and the kidney. In *Renal Disease,* 2nd ed. Ed. Black, D. A. K. Oxford: Blackwell.

Chapter 7

OBSTRUCTION

The filtration force at the glomerulus produces the glomerular filtrate and propels it through the renal tubules into the minor calyces of the kidney. Peristaltic waves of muscular contraction which start in the minor calyces and pass successively through the major calyces, the renal pelvis and the ureters, assisted to some extent by gravity, then propel urine into the bladder. The bladder stores urine and when some 300/400 ml have accumulated, contracts to expel it through the urethra.

Obstruction to the flow of urine, which is one of the common disturbances that urological surgeons are called upon to investigate and treat, is found most often at the pelvi-ureteric junction, in the ureter, at the neck of the bladder, or in the urethra.

The Effects of Obstruction

Stasis of urine

Obstruction causes back pressure and opposes the forces that produce urine at the glomerulus and propel it through the urinary tract. Urine accumulates and stagnates in those parts of the urinary tract that are above the obstruction.

Dilatation

The stagnant urine stretches and dilates the urinary tract above the level of obstruction. Obstruction at the pelvi-ureteric junction therefore causes dilatation of the pelvis and calyces of the kidney (hydronephrosis) (Fig. 24), while obstruction in the ureter causes dilatation of the ureter (hydroureter), and later of the pelvis and calyces also. Obstruction in the bladder neck or urethra causes dilatation of the bladder and later of both ureters and both renal pelves. Sometimes a diverticulum forms because a weak area of the bladder gives way (Fig. 25).

Dilatation stretches the muscle fibres of the urinary tract above the level of the obstruction, increasing their initial length

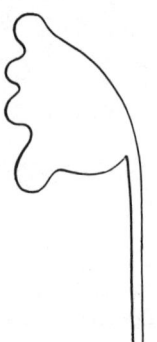

Fig. 24. Hydronephrosis.

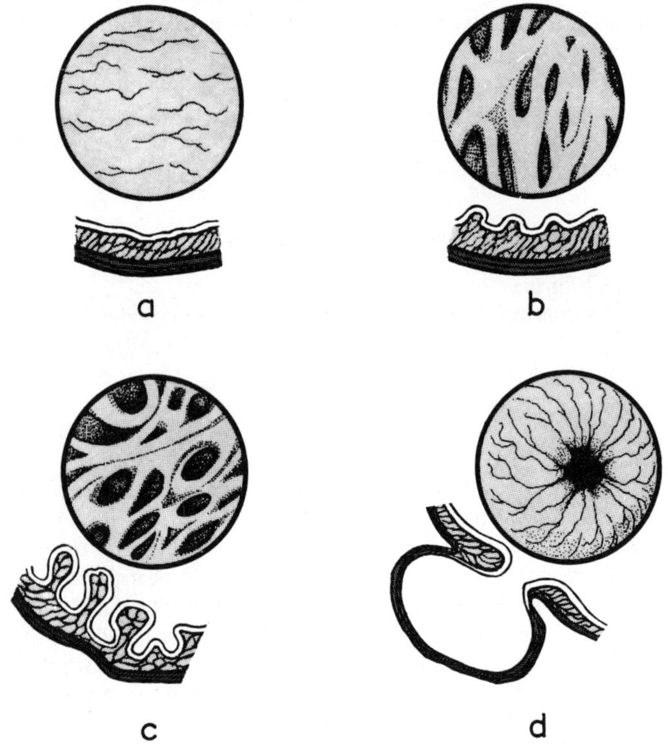

a

b

c

d

Fig. 25. Some effects of obstruction upon the bladder. a. Normal bladder. b. Early trabeculation. c. Severe trabeculation. d. Diverticulum.

and stimulating hypertrophy. At first they contract more strongly than normal, which helps to push urine through the obstructed segment. Stagnation is reduced but rarely eliminated entirely unless the degree of obstruction is minimal. Increasing dilatation overstretches and reduces the efficiency of the muscle fibres. Each part of the urinary tract tends to protect the parts above from the effects of obstruction; thus if the lower end of the ureter is obstructed, the lower third of the ureter dilates and only when it can no longer accommodate the accumulating urine is there successive dilatation of the middle and upper thirds of the ureter, pelvis and calyces (Fig. 26).

Interference with renal function

In the early stages of obstruction any reduction in renal function caused by back pressure is reversible if the obstruction is removed. As the pressure above the level of an obstruction increases, the pressure difference between the glomerulus and the

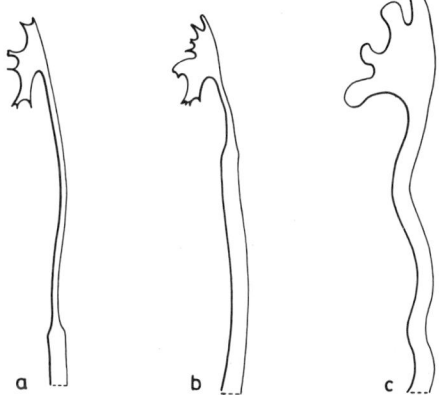

Fig. 26. Progressive dilatation of the ureter and renal pelvis when the lower end of the ureter is obstructed.

tubule, normally about 35 mm Hg, is reduced and so also are the rate and speed of glomerular filtration and the speed with which the filtrate travels through the tubules into the calyces. At first sight it might be expected that a completely obstructed kidney would cease functioning altogether. In fact, glomerular filtration rarely ceases completely even with complete obstruction. Although urine cannot pass down the ureter, small quantities

115

escape from the pelvis of the kidney into the veins, the lymphatics, the tubules or the interstices of the kidney by processes called respectively pyelo-venous, pyelo-lymphatic, pyelo-tubular and pyelo-interstitial backflow (Fig. 27). Backflow may allow some glomerular function to continue but does not, of course, enable the kidney to excrete waste products or to carry out its other functions. If a solitary kidney or if both kidneys are completely obstructed, the patient experiences acute renal failure, usually with anuria. Later the renal parenchyma and its

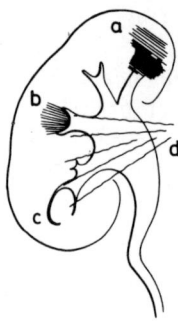

Fig. 27. Backflow. a. Pyelo-interstitial. b. Pyelo-tubular. c. Pyelo-venous. d. Pyelo-lymphatic.

blood supply are compressed by the dilating pelvis and calyces and further damaged by ischaemia, infection and stones. Renal failure caused by obstruction will always improve when the obstruction is removed, but how much it improves depends on how much parenchyma is damaged.

Infection and stones

The transitional epithelium lining the urinary tract is devoid of glands or hair follicles or other crevices in which organisms can hide. The flow of urine decontaminates the urinary tract of micro-organisms before they penetrate the wall of the urinary tract and cause infection, by washing them into and out of the bladder. Obstruction interferes with these natural defences and thus predisposes to infection and to stone formation (Fig. 28).

Neoplasms

Obstruction can predispose to neoplasia in two ways: (1) some transitional cell tumours are caused by carcinogenic agents in the

116

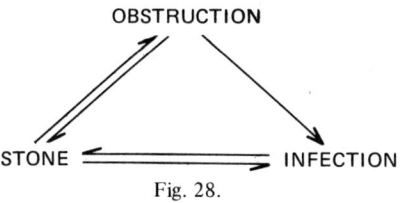

Fig. 28.

urine, which have more time to act if there is stagnation; (2) obstruction leads to infection and stone formation which induce metaplasia of transitional epithelium to squamous epithelium which may form squamous cell or epidermoid carcinomas.

Causes of Obstruction

Any lesion that narrows or interferes with peristalsis in the tubular parts of the urinary tract (that is, the necks of the calyces, the pelvi-ureteric junction, the ureters, the bladder neck and the urethra) may obstruct the flow of urine (Fig. 29). Such lesions may be classified as (a) lesions in the lumen, such as stone, blood clot or papilla; (b) lesions in the wall, such as strictures and tumours; (c) lesions outside the wall, such as an aberrant artery, fibrosis or tumour; (d) neuromuscular lesions. Neuromuscular lesions, which are usually congenital and which occur in the pelvi-ureteric junction or lower third of the ureter, do not narrow the lumen, but prevent the peristaltic wave and therefore urine from passing through.

If both ureters are obstructed the lesion is usually in or below the bladder. However, certain lesions may be extensive enough to involve both ureters above or behind the bladder (Fig. 30). The commonest of these is malignant disease that has spread from the prostate, cervix or bladder; but the fibrosis that follows X-ray treatment of carcinoma of the cervix or bladder, or pelvic operations or idiopathic retroperitoneal fibrosis may involve one or both ureters.

In idiopathic retroperitoneal fibrosis the retroperitoneal tissues are infiltrated by dense fibrous tissue, which may include a few chronic inflammatory cells. The fibrous tissue surrounds and compresses, but rarely infiltrates one or both ureters and most patients present with chronic renal failure. Sometimes it compresses the aorta or inferior vena cava thus obstructing the flow of blood into or out of the lower limbs, and it may be associated with constrictive pericarditis.

117

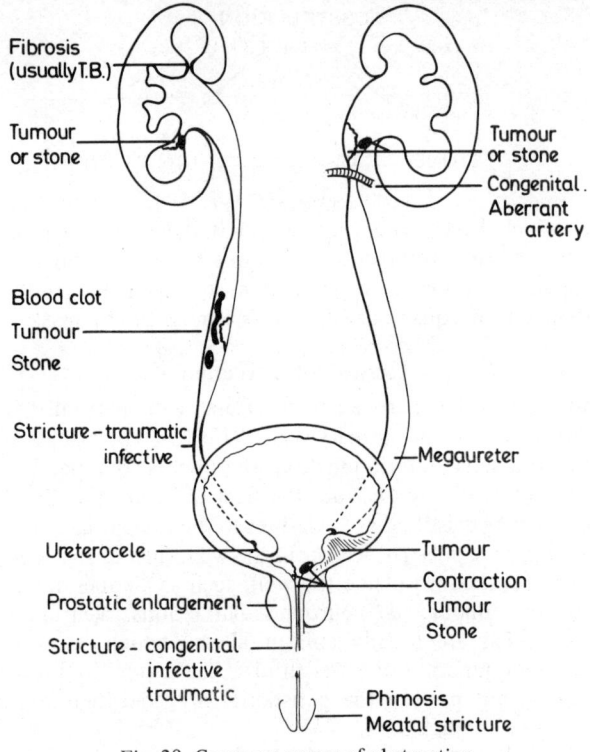

Fibrosis
(usually T.B.)

Tumour
or stone

Tumour
or stone

Congenital.
Aberrant
artery

Blood clot
Tumour
Stone

Stricture – traumatic
infective

Megaureter

Ureterocele

Tumour

Contraction
Tumour
Stone

Prostatic enlargement

Stricture - congenital
infective
traumatic

Phimosis
Meatal stricture

Fig. 29. Common causes of obstruction.

Although idiopathic retroperitoneal fibrosis has been variously attributed to low grade infection, to auto-immunity, to neoplastic change and to the effect of drugs like methersigide, its true cause remains a mystery, and to that extent it is similar to other fibrous conditions such as Peyronie's disease (p. 235) and Dupuytren's contracture.

Clinical Features of Obstruction

Although the effects of obstruction are similar whatever its level, the clinical features of obstruction above the bladder, and of obstruction below the bladder, are sufficiently different to be discussed separately.

Above bladder

Obstruction causes pain only if the kidney continues to

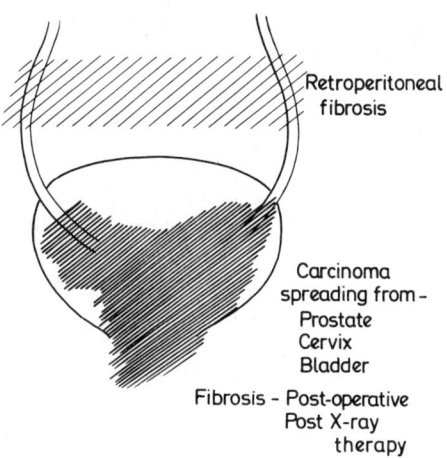

Retroperitoneal
fibrosis

Carcinoma
spreading from -
Prostate
Cervix
Bladder

Fibrosis - Post-operative
Post X-ray
therapy

Fig. 30. Lesions above or behind the bladder that may obstruct both ureters.

function. Because of backflow, it usually does so, even if the obstruction is complete. Sudden and almost complete obstruction (such as is caused by stone or blood clot) causes renal or ureteric colic. This is a severe sustained pain with exacerbations that starts in the loin and radiates to the front of the abdomen, iliac fossa, groin, thigh, scrotum or labia, and which is associated with nausea, vomiting, sweating and pallor. Moderate and gradual obstruction causes pain which is mild and which is often precipitated or aggravated by the diuresis that follows drinking.

Many patients present not with pain but with symptoms of the infection, the stones or the renal failure which obstruction may cause.

In an obstructed kidney infection can be severe because it is enclosed and because organisms can readily enter the blood stream by pyelo-venous or pyelo-lymphatic backflow. If organisms are unable to pass through the obstructon into the bladder, the urine remains sterile.

The patient may complain not only of symptoms caused by obstruction and its sequelae, but also of symptoms caused by the disease or lesion responsible for the obstruction.

Below bladder

The force and calibre of the urinary stream, the time taken for micturition and the completeness with which the bladder is

119

emptied, depend upon the balance between the force with which the bladder contracts and the resistance to be overcome in the neck of the bladder and urethra. The force and resistance are normally so balanced that the bladder is emptied quickly and completely each time urine is passed. When outflow obstruction increases the resistance, the force of bladder contraction gradually increases because the muscle fibres are stretched and hypertrophy. This compensation is incomplete unless obstruction is minimal, and the following conditions may result:

1. The patient has difficulty in starting micturition, the urinary stream is thin in calibre and poor in force, there is terminal dribbling, a feeling that the bladder is not completely emptied, and increased frequency of micturition especially at night.

2. Retention. Increasing obstruction will cause urinary retention which may be acute or chronic. In acute retention the patient is unable to pass urine despite an urgent desire to do so, and the bladder is tender, tense and distended. In chronic retention the bladder has gradually distended over a long period of time and small amounts of urine passively overflow at frequent intervals and with little control. The patient may be unaware that his bladder is distended and complain only of frequency and incontinence. The prolonged back pressure may already have caused bilateral hydronephrosis and hydroureter with chronic renal failure when the patient is first seen.

3. Chronic renal failure. Some patients may seek advice only when they have symptoms and signs of chronic renal failure.

4. The patient may present with other consequences of obstruction such as recurrent or chronic infections, or stones in the bladder or kidneys.

The relief of obstruction is necessary not only to preserve or restore renal function and to prevent stone formation, infection and neoplasm, but also to alleviate the patient's symptoms. Obstruction is relieved by treating the disease causing it but if this is impossible or has to be delayed, it may be temporarily relieved by draining the kidney (by nephrostomy), the ureter (by ureterostomy) or the bladder (by supra-pubic or urethral catheterization).

FURTHER READING

Bricker, N. S. (1963). In *Diseases of the Kidney*. Ed. Strauss, M. B. & Welt, L. G. London: Churchill.

Chapter 8

INFECTIONS OF THE URINARY TRACT

Perinephric Abscess

The perinephric fat lies between the renal capsule and the renal fascia and surrounds the kidney. It may be infected by organisms which spread directly into it from some infection of the kidney, but is more often infected by staphylococci carried by the blood stream from a distant focus such as a boil or carbuncle of the skin while the kidney itself is normal. Because a perinephric abscess is deeply situated and surrounded by thick muscles and viscera, it is often large before it produces such local signs as tenderness, swelling and redness. Fever, sometimes with rigors, malaise and vague loin pain, leucocytosis and a high erythrocyte sedimentation rate are the early symptoms and signs. A valuable physical sign is flattening of the normal concavity of the loin, which is most easily detected by looking down the back of the sitting patient. An X-ray of the abdomen may show downward displacement of the kidney, upward displacement and fixation of the diaphragm, and a soft-tissue shadow which obliterates the outline of the psoas muscle.

A perinephric abscess can be distinguished from acute pyelonephritis which also causes fever, and pain and tenderness in the loin, because it rarely communicates with the kidney and therefore the urine contains neither pus nor organisms, and there is no associated cystitis or disturbance of micturition.

By the time that perinephric infection is diagnosed it has usually progressed to abscess formation and the abscess should be incised through a lumbar incision and drained.

Low grade non-suppurative inflammation may occur in the perinephric fat and is often found in association with calculi, or non-specific or tuberculous infections of the kidney. As the result of such inflammation, the perinephric fat becomes adherent to the capsule or pelvis of the kidney, making operations on that organ more difficult than usual.

Renal Abscess or Carbuncle

A localized abscess or carbuncle in the renal parenchyma is, like perinephric abscess, usually caused by staphylococci carried by the blood stream from a distant focus. It is usually solitary and situated in the renal cortex. Because it rarely spreads into the calyces or pelvis of the kidney, it is unusual for pus or organisms to appear in the urine or for the patient to have any disturbance of micturition.

The clinical features of renal abscess are similar to those of perinephric abscess, but do not include swelling in the loin unless the infection spreads into the perinephric fat. A renal abscess distorts and displaces the calyces and even the pelvis of the kidney, and appears in pyelograms as a space-occupying lesion, but is seldom large enough to obliterate the psoas shadow. Most renal abscesses resolve with antibiotic therapy, but some have to be incised and drained.

In pyaemic conditions such as bacterial endocarditis and in some severe cases of acute pyelonephritis, multiple small abscesses appear in the kidney. In pyaemia, the abscesses develop from septic emboli in the smaller renal blood vessels and therefore appear first in the glomeruli. In acute pyelonephritis, on the other hand, infection spreads into the parenchyma from the renal pelvis, and abscesses appear first in the renal medulla.

PYELONEPHRITIS AND CYSTITIS

The term urinary tract infections usually implies pyelonephritis or cystitis. The two are often associated because micro-organisms can readily ascend from the bladder to the kidney, or descend from the kidney to the bladder.

Pyelonephritis

Pyelonephritis is caused by micro-organisms which invade the pelvis and parenchyma of one or both kidneys and the inflammatory changes are focal and irregular, and most marked in the medulla. Unlike pyelonephritis, glomerulonephritis is not infective, is diffuse and symmetrical throughout both kidneys, and primarily affects the renal cortex.

122

Aetiology. In first attacks of pyelonephritis, the micro-organism responsible is usually a coliform like *E. coli,* but is sometimes *Proteus mirabilis, Klebsiella aerogenes, Streptococcus faecalis* or *Staphylococcus aureus.* In chronic or recurrent infections, although the same micro-organisms are found they are often associated with others such as *Proteus vulgaris* and pseudomonas, especially if the urinary tract contains stone or the infection follows operation or urethral instrumentation. (Tuberculous infections of the urinary tract are considered on p. 136.)

Route and source of infection. Normally, the anterior urethra contains micro-organisms, whereas the posterior urethra and the urinary tract proximal to it are sterile. The fact that the urethral mucosa has antibacterial properties and is frequently washed with sterile urine discourages the spread of organisms from the anterior urethra to the bladder and ureters. Because the female urethra is short, wide and straight, organisms can pass more easily along it than along the male urethra and urinary infections are much commoner in females than in males.

Organisms can reach the kidneys not only by retrograde spread along the ureters, but also by the blood stream or by the lymphatics, although there is little evidence to support lymphatic spread. Experimental work on animals suggests that the haematogenous route is particularly important if a kidney is obstructed. Some blood-borne infections predominantly affect the medulla because it has a poorer blood supply and a higher osmotic pressure than the cortex. In man, however, of the organisms that cause renal infections, only staphylococci spread by way of the blood stream and they affect the cortex more than the medulla and cause solitary or multiple renal abscesses rather than pyelonephritis. It is considered that in most cases of pyelonephritis in humans the organisms ascend along the ureters from the lower urinary tract. The normal urinary tract can decontaminate itself of micro-organisms before they cause infection by means of (a) the flow of urine which washes organisms down before they have a chance to invade the mucosa and (b) the smooth nature of the transitional epithelium which contains no hair follicles, sweat glands or other crevices in which organisms can hide and so escape the flow of urine. Many think that these defence mechanisms have little, if any, value yet they believe that washing the skin of the hands, which contains many glands and hair

123

follicles in which organisms can hide, is a reasonably effective, though temporary, way of decontaminating them. Although acute and chronic pyelonephritis can occur in patients with normal urinary tracts, more often than not there is a predisposing abnormality.

Abnormalities which predispose to pyelonephritis

Obstruction. Obstruction to the free flow of urine interferes with the ability of the kidney and the urinary tract to decontaminate themselves of organisms before they cause infection. Furthermore, obstruction to the bladder is frequently associated with vesico-ureteric reflux, which enables organisms to ascend from the lower urinary tract to the kidneys, and with diverticulum formation.

Pregnancy. Hydroureter and hydronephrosis, most marked on the right side, always occur during pregnancy and persist for some months afterwards. The dilatation is attributed partly to muscular relaxation caused by high progesterone levels, and partly to obstruction of the ureters by the pregnant uterus.

Systemic disease. Diabetes, leukaemia and myxoedema all reduce the resistance of the body to infection and therefore predispose to urinary tract infections.

Stones. Stones predispose to infection not only by causing obstruction and stasis but also by damaging the epithelial lining of the urinary tract.

Phenacetin. Phenacetin alone may cause chronic interstitial nephritis, but it also predisposes the kidney to infection.

Neurological abnormalities. Some nervous diseases interfere with micturition and the residuum of urine that remains in the bladder after micturition predisposes to infection.

Fistulae. Fistulae between the bladder and the colon tend to produce urinary tract infections because colonic organisms enter the bladder and may ascend to the kidneys.

Foreign bodies. Foreign bodies in the urinary tract, especially ones that communicate with the exterior, like drainage or nephrostomy tubes, urethral or supra-pubic catheters, predispose to infection, and it is impossible to eradicate the infection so long as the foreign body remains.

Vesico-ureteric reflux. Normally all the urine contained in the bladder is expelled through the urethra on micturition. X-rays taken during micturition after the instillation of radio-opaque dye into the bladder, show that, in some people, urine passes up the ureters as well as out through the urethra. This abnormality is called vesico-ureteric reflux, and it may be primary or secondary.

Primary vesico-ureteric reflux occurs in a urinary tract which is apparently normal and it is more common than is supposed. It can be demonstrated in a high proportion of patients, especially infants with recurrent urinary tract infections, and it appears to be the mechanism by which organisms ascend to the kidneys in most cases of pyelonephritis in which there is no other apparent predisposing cause. However, some believe that reflux is the result and not the cause of infection, and there is evidence to support this because reflux often disappears when the infection is eradicated by antibiotics.

Secondary vesico-urteric reflux frequently occurs if the outflow tract from the bladder is obstructed, if there is a bladder diverticulum near a ureteric orifice or if micturition is disturbed by nervous lesions.

Sexual trauma in the female. Sexual intercourse may injure the female urethra which lies close to the vagina, or milk organisms along it into the bladder and cause infections, sometimes severe, of the bladder or kidney or both.

Instrumentation. Infection may be introduced into the bladder or kidney or existing infections may be exacerbated by urethral and ureteric catheterization, cystoscopy and other endoscopic procedures, especially if they are carried out in obstructed or infected bladders. Ascending pyelonephritis with septicaemia is a not uncommon sequel and used to be called 'catheter fever'.

Acute Pyelonephritis

Pathology

The kidney is swollen and soft. The pelvis and calyces contain purulent urine which may be blood-stained and their mucosal lining is congested and oedematous. The renal medulla is infiltrated by many neutrophil polymorphs, and a few lymphocytes and plasma cells. Later the cortex is involved as inflammatory cells spread through the tubules and the interstitial spaces between them, but the glomeruli are rarely involved. In severe infections linear abscesses appear in both medulla and cortex. Pyelonephritis is a focal condition and areas of normal kidney are found among areas of inflammation.

Clinical features

The clinical features of acute pyelonephritis are usually characteristic. In about 9 cases out of 10, the patient is a woman. There is an abrupt onset with fever, malaise, nausea, vomiting and pain in the loin or hypochondrium. Frequency of micturition, dysuria and sometimes strangury occur because the bladder is irritated by infected urine or is inflamed. Children with acute pyelonephritis do not always complain of frequency and dysuria, although fever may be severe enough to cause convulsions and the child may scream during micturition because of pain. The urine should be examined for pus cells and organisms in all children with unexplained pyrexia.

In acute pyelonephritis the urine contains organisms, pus cells and sometimes blood. The urine is acid if the organisms are coliforms, alkaline if they are proteus which can split urea to ammonia. The urinary deposit may contain fragments of renal papillae if necrotizing papillitis complicates the infection, as sometimes occurs in phenacetin nephropathy and diabetes. Leucocytosis occurs and the erythrocyte sedimentation rate is elevated. The blood pressure and blood urea levels are usually normal, but if much fluid is lost by sweating or vomiting or if both kidneys are infected, the blood urea may be elevated and the urine output reduced.

Organisms can pass from the pelvis of the kidney into the blood stream by pyelo-venous or pyelo-lymphatic backflow. They may be rapidly destroyed causing no more than a transient bacteraemia but sometimes they survive and proliferate, causing septicaemia. If acute pyelonephritis is bilateral or associated with septicaemia the patient is severely ill, with high fever, rigors, severe oliguria and sometimes shock. Blood cultures must be taken from all patients who have pyelonephritis with a severe systemic disturbance. If an obstructed kidney becomes acutely infected it is enlarged, tender and usually palpable. Unless obstruction is relieved, infection may progress to a pyonephrosis, in which the dilated pelvis and calyces are filled with pus. A pyonephrosis is unlikely to resolve with antibiotics alone and may have to be drained by a nephrostomy tube or even removed.

Treatment

First attack

Approximately 90 per cent of first attack cases of acute

126

pyelonephritis occurring outside a hospital are caused by sulphonamide-sensitive *E. coli.* A substantial proportion of the remainder are caused by *Proteus mirabilis* or *Klebsiella aerogenes,* which may also respond to sulphonamides. To treat such first attack cases with sulphonamides, such as Sulphadimidine 500 mg thrice daily for 7 days, is reasonable. Although Sulphadimidine is more soluble than many other sulphonamides, it is still advisable to ensure a high fluid intake in order to prevent the deposition of sulphonamide crystals in the tubules.

Sulphonamides are bacteriostatic rather than bactericidal, and pus interferes with their action, and if extensive tissue damage or bacteraemia is suspected, a bactericidal agent like Ampicillin should be given until the result of bacteriological examination of the urine is available.

Sulphonamides may suppress the symptoms of pyelonephritis without effecting a cure, and it is very important to send a mid-stream specimen of urine for culture a week or two after the cessation of therapy.

Recurrent pyelonephritis

The recurrence of acute pyelonephritis suggests that the initial infection has not been eradicated, or that there is a predisposing cause which continues to operate. Previous antibiotic therapy may have altered the nature and the sensitivity of the bacterial flora. Most patients referred to hospital with pyelonephritis are recurrent cases, and in only 50 per cent of them are the micro-organisms sensitive to sulphonamides. Acute pyelonephritis that occurs in obstructed kidneys, or follows instrumentation, or operation, is often severe and is usually caused by *Proteus vulgaris, Pseudomonas pyocyaneus,* or antibiotic-resistant strains of *E. coli.* Sulphonamides are not the drugs of choice in recurrent or complicated causes of pyelonephritis. Both blood and urine cultures should be obtained before any antibiotic is given, unless the patient is severely ill, when a bactericidal antibiotic such as Ampicillin or Kanamycin may be used.

All patients with recurrent acute pyelonephritis must be carefully investigated in order to identify and if possible treat any predisposing cause.

Chronic Pyelonephritis

Aetiology

Many believe that chronic pyelonephritis develops from

recurrent or inadequately treated acute pyelonephritis, because two-thirds of patients say or admit on direct questioning that they have had frequency and dysuria at some time in the past. However, many patients with recurrent acute pyelonephritis never develop established chronic pyelonephritis, and only 20 per cent of patients with established chronic pyelonephritis have positive urine cultures. Furthermore, although acute pyelonephritis occurs 10 times as often in females as in males, established chronic pyelonephritis is found as often in males as in females. In many patients with obstructive lesions of the urinary tract, the transition from acute to chronic pyelonephritis can often be readily traced.

Pathology

Unlike glomerulonephritis, chronic pyelonephritis is focal and irregular. It may be unilateral or bilateral, but when both kidneys are involved one is usually more severely affected than the other. At first, the kidney is macroscopically normal, but progressive fibrosis and scarring gradually destroy the parenchyma and eventually the kidney becomes small, granular and contracted. The small fibrosed kidney of chronic pyelonephritis is similar to the contracted kidney seen in the end stages of glomerulonephritis. However, in pyelonephritis, the renal papillae are destroyed in the scarred areas of the medulla, and the calyces are dilated which produces a characteristic appearance on pyelography called 'clubbing'.

The inflammatory cells are mainly lymphocytes, monocytes and plasma cells. They invade the renal pelvis and spread into the medulla between and through the tubules, which may be so damaged that they can be recognized only with difficulty. Obstruction and obliteration of the distal nephron causes dilatation of the proximal tubules and hyaline casts form in the stagnant urine they contain. The dilated tubules look like thyroid acini and the term 'thyroid change' is used to describe them. At first, the glomeruli are little affected, but eventually inflammatory cells break through Bowman's capsule and involve the glomeruli. The glomeruli are also damaged by ischaemia, because interstitial fibrosis and hypertension, if they develop, gradually occlude the glomerular capillaries.

The most characteristic histological lesion of chronic pyelonephritis is sometimes called chronic interstitial nephritis and is inflammation and fibrosis of the interstitial spaces between the tubules. Chronic interstitial nephritis, however, occurs from many causes other than infection, particularly ischaemia, analgesics, irradiation, gout and hypercalcaemia.

Clinical features

Chronic pyelonephritis may present in a number of ways:

1. As recurrent acute pyelonephritis. Acute pyelonephritis tends to recur, sometimes many times. A few patients with recurrent acute pyelonephritis develop the functional, radiological and pathological changes of chronic pyelonephritis, but many do not.

2. As asymptomatic bacteriuria. Many females, both children and adults, are found to have significant numbers of organisms in their urine despite the absence of symptoms of any kind. No less than 1.2 per cent of normal schoolgirls have asymptomatic bacteriuria whereas the incidence in schoolboys is only 0.2 per cent. Only a few patients with asymptomatic bacteriuria have radiological evidence of chronic pyelonephritis. Nevertheless it is generally accepted that a bacterial count of 10^5 or more in a properly collected midstream specimen of urine indicates active infection of the kidneys or bladder or both, even if there is neither clinical nor radiological evidence of infection.

3. With mild frequency, mild dysuria and sometimes loin pain. These are perhaps the commonest symptoms of chronic pyelonephritis, but they are sometimes so vague and indefinite as to be of little diagnostic help. Nevertheless, they should stimulate a search for urinary infection, which can be diagnosed with confidence only if there is significant bacteriuria. General malaise and vague ill-health and other common and indefinite symptoms should not be attributed to chronic pyelonephritis unless urine cultures are positive or the radiological findings are definite.

4. With impaired renal function. Almost half the patients with chronic pyelonephritis have a significant impairment of renal function. Sometimes both glomerular and tubular function are equally impaired, and the clinical picture is indistinguishable from that of chronic glomerulonephritis except that proteinuria is never massive and often remarkably slight. About one quarter of the patients with renal failure have hypertension, and it may be of the malignant variety. Usually, however, tubular function is disproportionately reduced, and patients have normal glomerular filtration rates but severe impairment of concentrating ability and

therefore polyuria. That the medulla bears the brunt of chronic pyelonephritis explains the preponderance of tubular dysfunction in these patients. Less common than loss of concentrating ability alone, are acquired tubular acidosis, salt-wasting conditions, and acquired nephrogenic diabetes insipidus.

Diagnosis

In a few patients there is clear evidence of progression from recurrent acute pyelonephritis with normal renal function to established chronic pyelonephritis with renal impairment. In many patients, however, chronic pyelonephritis is by no means easy to diagnose.

Symptoms. Frequency, dysuria, loin pain and vague ill-health may not be prominent features of the patient's illness, and even when present do not necessarily indicate infection.

Examination of the urine A bacterial count of 10^5 organisms per ml in a carefully collected midstream specimen of urine is accepted as indicating active infection in either the kidneys or the bladder. An increased excretion of white cells indicates inflammation, but not necessarily infection.

Agglutination tests. Although a high serum agglutination titre against an infecting organism suggests tissue invasion, the place of such tests in the diagnosis of pyelonephritis has not yet been firmly established, but they may become more prominent in the future.

Radiological evidence (Fig. 31). The demonstration of certain characteristic changes on pyelography suggests chronic pyelonephritis, especially if these changes are accompanied by bacteriological evidence of past or present infection. The end result of pyelonephritis is a wedge-shaped scar which involves the whole thickness of the kidney, although the medulla is more involved than the cortex. In the scarred area the papillae are destroyed and the calyx is dilated or clubbed. Pyelonephritis is focal and the scarring is irregularly distributed. If both kidneys are affected, one is usually more severely involved than the other. X-rays may also reveal obstruction or some other predisposing cause for the infection. Vesico-ureteric reflux may be demonstrated in a micturating cystogram.

Renal biopsy. This is of little value in the diagnosis of chronic pyelonephritis. Pyelonephritis is a focal disease, and the tissue obtained may be normal despite severe changes in other parts of

130

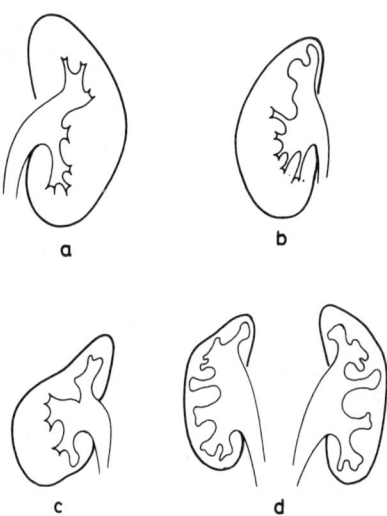

Fig. 31. The effects of chronic pyelonephritis on the kidney. a. Normal. b. Scarring in upper pole. c. Scarring in upper and lower poles. d. Diffuse bilateral scarring.

the kidney. Even a biopsy sample showing interstitial nephritis is of limited diagnostic value, because these changes occur from causes other than infection. The most characteristic pathological changes of chronic pyelonephritis are in the calyces, and calyceal tissue is not, or should not, be obtained by percutaneous renal biopsy.

Renal function tests. Overall impairment of renal function can occur in almost any renal disease. Chronic pyelonephritis, unlike glomerulonephritis, impairs tubular more than glomerular function. The demonstration of severe impairment in the ability of the kidney to concentrate or acidify the urine in the presence of a relatively normal glomerular filtration rate suggests chronic pyelonephritis, but is far from diagnostic.

Comment

The difficulty in diagnosing chronic pyelonephritis is real. Only about 20 per cent of so-called 'established cases' give positive urine cultures, and unequivocal radiological evidence, but what is an 'established case'? In one series of over 3,000 autopsies, chronic pyelonephritis was diagnosed in 3 per cent of cases. In another smaller autopsy series, the incidence was 17 per cent. Many agents other than micro-organisms produce chronic interstitial nephritis, and to regard infection as the cause in all chronically inflamed kidneys is a mistake. Even the demonstration of bacterial invasion is not proof that pyelonephritis is the primary disease because scarred renal tissue is liable to be secondarily infected, whatever the cause of the scarring. Chronic pyelonephritis was first described in 1917, but it was not until 1940 that it became recognized as an important and common disease entity. Now we tend to clutch at the flimsiest straw of evidence that provides an excuse for making the diagnosis, and the natural history of pyelonephritis and the effect of therapy will not become clear until uniform and critical diagnostic criteria become established.

Treatment

All patients with chronic pyelonephritis must be carefully investigated with a view to identifying and, where possible, removing the predisposing cause. In some patients, the treatment of chronic pyelonephritis is that of chronic renal failure, as discussed in Chapter 4. Continuing infection will cause or hasten the decline in renal function, and to identify the responsible organism if at all possible and to give the appropriate antibiotic is obviously important. Infection tends to recur, and regular checks on the urine for evidence of bacterial growth must be made. Some centres give short, intensive courses of antibiotics whenever there is a recrudescence of infection, whereas others give a short course of intensive therapy followed by a prolonged course of low dosage 'suppressive' antibiotic treatment. There is no evidence yet that indicates which method yields the best results.

Choice of antibacterial agent

Sulphonamides. In recent years, the serious side effects of sulphonamides have been stressed but if the vast amount prescribed is considered it seems unlikely that they are any more dangerous than many other antibacterial agents. Sulphonamides are bacteriostatic. They arrest bacterial multiplication, but leave the task of eradicating the infection to the body's own defences, and should be used only in first attack, uncomplicated acute pyelonephritis.

Sulphonamides with trimethoprim. Trimethoprim, like the

132

sulphonamides, is bacteriostatic, but when used together, these two agents act synergistically and have a bactericidal effect. 'Septrin' tablets each contain 80 mg of trimethoprim and 400 mg of sulphamethoxazole, and the dose is 4 tablets daily. Sulphonamide/trimethoprim combinations should not be given to pregnant women, as tetrogenic effects have been noted in rats, nor to patients receiving folic acid antagonists for immuno-suppression or for the treatment of malignant disease, because they may potentiate the action of such drugs.

Penicillin group. *Ampicillin.* This synthetic penicillin is active against many Gram-negative organisms, including *E. coli* and *Proteus mirabilis,* but is useless against penicillinase-producing organisms. If there is much damage to renal tissue, conventional oral dosage may not produce adequate tissue levels in the infected areas. Although more liable than many other antibiotics to cause skin rashes and gastro-intestinal side effects, it is a useful drug for acute and recurrent infections of the kidney and the bladder.

Carbenecillin. This synthetic penicillin is of particular interest because it is active against pseudomonas. It is less effective against this organism than either the polymixins or gentamicin, but has fewer side effects.

Cephalosporins. Cephalosporins have a wide antibacterial spectrum. They are active against a considerable number of Gram-positive and Gram-negative organisms, but not against pseudomonas. The most widely used of these agents is Cephaloridine, which must be given by injection, although a new preparation known as Cephaloxin has been introduced and is suitable for oral use. Cephalosporins should be reserved for severe infections, because they are expensive and sometimes cause nephropathy.

Tetracyclines. These wide spectrum drugs are bacteriostatic and effective against *E. coli*. They are deposited in developing teeth and bone, and therefore are contra-indicated in pregnant women and in children.

Chloramphenicol. Because this drug is relatively expensive, carries a significant risk of marrow depression and is excreted in the urine mainly in the form of inactive metabolites, it has little, if any, place in the treatment of urinary tract infections.

Aminoglycosides. This group of antibacterial drugs includes streptomycin, kanamycin, neomycin and gentamicin. All have similar pharmacological effects, must be given parenterally and can irreversibly damage the eighth nerve. They are excreted unchanged in the urine and accumulate in the body if there is renal failure. Renal function must be assessed before they are given, and if it is impaired, dosage of aminoglycosides must be carefully controlled by estimating blood levels.

Streptomycin is rarely employed in urinary tract infections because organisms rapidly become resistant to it.

Neomycin is too toxic for systemic use.

Kanamycin is active against most organisms found in urinary tract infections, except *Streptococcus faecalis* and pseudomonas. It has nephrotoxic actions which are reversible and ototoxic actions which are not. Nevertheless, it is probably the drug of choice in serious infections, especially when they are complicated by septicaemia.

Gentamicin has recently become available and is effective against pseudomonas. Eighth nerve damage occurs at blood levels of 10 μg per ml or over, whereas streptomycin and kanamycin have this effect at blood levels of 30 μg per ml or more.

Polymixins. These rather toxic antibiotics are effective against a wide range of Gram-negative organisms, including pseudomonas. There is little to choose between polymixin B and polymixin E (Colomycin).

Nalidixic acid (Negram). This is taken orally and is effective against many Gram-negative organisms: klebsiella, proteus and some hospital strains of *E. coli* resistant to other oral antibiotics are often sensitive to it. Bacteria soon acquire resistance to it, however, and so it is of little use in long-term therapy.

Nitrofurantoin. This is a synthetic drug active against many bacteria, but is of little value in systemic infections because effective blood levels often cause intolerable nausea and vomiting. However, high urine concentrations can be attained with small doses if renal function is good. It is effective against most strains of *E. coli* found in domiciliary practice, and is as useful as the sulphonamides or ampicillin for the treatment of bacteriuria during pregnancy. In renal failure small doses may produce high blood levels, and cause neuropathy.

134

Cycloserine. This is effective against many sulphonamide-resistant strains of *E. coli*. It is concentrated in the urine if renal function is normal and is of value as a long-term suppressant of recurrent infection when given in low doses. It should not be given if the blood urea level is even slightly raised because urine levels become ineffective, and tissue levels rise, causing serious side effects.

Hexamine and mandelic acid. These agents are usually given together orally in the form of Mandelamine (hexamine mandelate). Mandelic acid and formaldehyde are released in the acid urine, and both have antibacterial effects, but not against proteus. In renal failure Mandelamine is of little use because the urine cannot be made acid. Organisms rarely develop resistance to Mandelamine and it has a place in the treatment of intractable infections which have become resistant to other agents.

Alteration of urinary pH

Alteration of urinary pH may potentiate antibiotics. Sulphonamides and the amino-glucosides are more active in alkaline media, whereas tetracyclines, Cycloserine and Mandelamine are more active in acid media.

In *E. coli* infections the urine is acid and alkaline salts alone, like sodium bicarbonate or potassium citrate or both, may relieve symptoms.

In proteus infections the urine is alkaline, but salts like ammonium chloride are of little value because the alkalinity is caused by the splitting of urea in the urinary tract.

High fluid intake

In all patients with urinary tract infections, the patient is usually encouraged to drink in the hope of potentiating the flushing action of urine, which is one of the main natural decontaminating mechanisms of the urinary tract. Some believe that a high fluid intake merely dilutes the urinary concentration of antibacterial agents and therefore is harmful.

Cystitis

Inflammation of the bladder is called cystitis and may be acute or chronic.

Acute Cystitis

Acute cystitis is caused by the same types of organisms as are responsible for acute pyelonephritis. They reach the bladder usually by ascending along the urethra, unless the cystitis is secondary to pyelonephritis when they descend from the kidney. Cystitis, like pyelonephritis, is usually secondary to some predisposing cause such as urethral instrumentation, obstruction, stone, foreign body, or, in the female, sexual intercourse.

Clinical features

The onset, often preceded by instrumentation or intercourse, is acute. There is a marked increase in the frequency of micturition, dysuria, urgency, and sometimes strangury and haematuria, which may be severe. If haematuria is a prominent feature, the infection is called acute haemorrhagic cystitis. Acute cystitis has many features in common with acute pyelonephritis and indeed the two conditions may occur at the same time because organisms can easily travel from bladder to kidney or from kidney to bladder. In cystitis, urinary symptoms are severe and systemic disturbance is mild or even absent, whereas in acute pyelonephritis systemic symptoms are marked and urinary symptoms usually mild.

Like acute pyelonephritis, acute cystitis tends to recur if the predisposing cause continues to operate.

Chronic Cystitis

This is always associated with some predisposing cause such as obstruction, stone, fistula, foreign body or neurological disorder. The chief symptoms are increased frequency of micturition, dysuria and urgency. Tuberculosis and several non-infective bladder disorders cause symptoms indistinguishable from those of chronic cystitis, and are discussed later.

TUBERCULOSIS OF THE KIDNEYS AND URINARY TRACT

Urinary tuberculosis always starts in the kidney and is always secondary to tuberculosis elsewhere in the body, usually in the

136

lungs, but it may present long after the primary focus has healed. In many, if not all, patients with renal tuberculosis, both kidneys are involved, although one kidney is always worse than the other.

Pathology

The initial lesion in tuberculosis of the urinary tract is a minute cortical focus in the kidney, caused by organisms which have spread by the blood stream. Infection spreads through the tubules and through the interstitial tissues, and the pyramids and papillae are soon infected. Tuberculous follicles in a papilla coalesce and later burst into the related calyx. Pus and debris enter the renal pelvis, which also becomes involved.

The course of tuberculosis fluctuates even without treatment, and calcification, which is visible radiologically, occurs in the infected areas.

Tuberculosis of the ureters or bladder is always secondary to renal tuberculosis. Tubercle bacilli spread into the renal pelvis and down the ureter into the bladder as soon as a renal focus ulcerates into a calyx. If the entire ureter is involved, it thickens, fibroses and adheres to the retroperitoneal tissues. More often, only the lower third of the ureter is involved, and as fibrosis occurs, a stricture forms which obstructs the flow of urine down the ureter and leads to hydroureter and hydronephrosis.

In the bladder, tubercle bacilli cause congestion and oedema and small tubercles appear around the ureteric orifice. Later, ulceration and fibrosis occur, and spread to involve the entire bladder. As the bladder contracts, the affected ureteric orifice is distorted and drawn up and sometimes is called a 'golfhole orifice'.

Clinical features

The symptoms of urinary tuberculosis are similar to those of chronic pyelonephritis. The earliest symptom is increased frequency of micturition. Haematuria is inconsistent and often transient. The urine is usually acid and contains pus cells. The tubercle bacillus does not grow on ordinary culture, and the urine will be apparently sterile unless secondary infection has occurred with coliforms, proteus or pseudomonas. Such secondary infections are common, but seldom severe.

Diagnosis

X-rays

Plain X-rays may reveal calcified areas in one or both kidneys.

Intravenous pyelography may show no abnormality in the early stages of the disease. However, once infection has spread to involve a calyx, that calyx loses its clear-cut outline and becomes shaggy and clubbed, often communicating with an abscess cavity in the medulla and cortex. As the disease progresses more calyces are involved and large, irregular cavities form. Extensive cavitation may be followed by spontaneous healing, and the kidney becomes completely calcified. The ureters appear normal in the early stages of the disease but soon become irregular and rigid, and occasionally have a beaded appearance. If a stricture forms at the lower end of a ureter, the ureter, the pelvis and the calyces above, dilate, and renal function is reduced not only by cavitation and destruction but also by obstruction.

Cystoscopy

In the bladder, the earliest lesions appear around the ureteric orifice, where oedema, congestion and later small tubercles can be seen. Later, congestion and oedema may involve the whole of the bladder and tuberculous ulcers appear. With increasing fibrosis, the bladder capacity becomes progressively reduced, and may ultimately be as little as 25 ml.

Bacteriology

Even in established cases of urinary tract tuberculosis, the number of organisms present in the urine tends to be small in comparison with the numbers found in other bacterial infections. For this reason, an ordinary midstream specimen is not suitable for the diagnosis of tuberculosis, and at least three early morning specimens of urine must be sent to the laboratory. The centrifuged deposit of the urine is stained by the Ziehl-Neelsen method and examined for acid-fast bacilli. Smegma bacilli are also acid-fast, and diagnosis depends on culture. For culture of the tubercle bacillus, the centrifuged deposit is inoculated on to Lowenstein-Jensen medium. A culture cannot be regarded as negative until incubation has continued for at least 6 weeks. Guinea-pig inoculation was a widely used method in the past. It is more troublesome than Lowenstein-Jensen culture, and many guinea-pigs have a degree of resistance to tuberculosis and give false negative results.

138

In urinary tuberculosis, midstream urines are usually sterile. Secondary infection with coliforms or proteus occasionally occur, however, and cases of tuberculosis have been missed because the patient's symptoms are attributed to these secondary invaders. If there are grounds for suspecting tuberculosis, three early morning specimens of urine should be obtained regardless of the results obtained on ordinary culture. Secondary infection should not be treated with drugs possessing antituberculous activity, because such therapy obscures the diagnosis and may lead to the development of resistance to the drug employed for the tubercle bacillus.

GENITAL TUBERCULOSIS

In 50 per cent of patients with tuberculosis of the genital tract, the urinary tract also is involved, and a full urological examination must be carried out in all patients with genital tuberculosis.

Tuberculous epididymitis

Tubercle bacilli spread to the epididymis from the seminal vesicles or prostate by way of the vas deferens. The tail of the epididymis is the first part to be involved. Early lesions can be recognized as numerous hard, irregular nodules, which are usually described as craggy. The lesions progress to involve the whole epididymis, which may enlarge to 4 or 5 times its normal size. The caseating lesions may liquefy, forming cold abscesses, and the overlying skin becomes dusky, shiny and adherent to the underlying epididymis. An abscess may rupture through the skin and form a persistent sinus which discharges yellow inoffensive pus from which tubercle bacilli can be cultured.

Tuberculous prostatitis

Tubercle bacilli can infect the prostate by spreading from the bladder or by way of the blood stream. The gland enlarges and becomes irregular and craggy in consistence. In X-rays of the pelvis, areas of calcification can usually be seen within the gland.

Tuberculous infection of the seminal vesicles

Normal seminal vesicles are not palpable on rectal examination, but seminal vesicles affected by tuberculosis may enlarge to

4 or 5 times their normal size and become palpable. Calcification of the vesicles occurs, and this can often be seen as a 'butterfly-wing opacity' in X-rays of the pelvis.

Treatment of Urinary and Genital Tuberculosis

Chemotherapy will eradicate tuberculous infection provided that two or more drugs to which the organism is sensitive are given for a period of about 2 years. The three standard drugs are Isoniazid (200-400 mg/day), para-amino-salicylic acid (10–15 g/day) and streptomycin (0.75 to 1.0 g/day). Streptomycin is often omitted because it has to be given by injection and has side effects involving the eighth nerve. Even when infection is controlled, fibrosis may continue and cause strictures in the necks of the calyces, renal pelvis or ureter, or contraction of the bladder. Fibrosis can be discouraged with cortico-steroids such as Prednisolone in a dosage of 10 to 20 mg/day, and are often given along with the other drugs.

If the tubercle bacilli are resistant to two or more of the three first line drugs, second line drugs such as pyrizinamide, ethionamide, cycloserine or rifampicin may be required. All these drugs have toxic side effects and must be given only under careful supervision.

Surgery

Most patients with urinary or genital tuberculosis are cured by chemotherapy alone. Some require surgery. Surgery does not replace chemotherapy unless the bacilli are resistant to both the first and the second line drugs, but is sometimes required to alleviate the effects of fibrosis in kidney, ureter or bladder. The progress of the disease is assessed by pyelography at 3- or 6-monthly intervals during treatment, and a decision to carry out surgery is rarely made until 3 months, and sometimes not until 18 or even 24 months after chemotherapy starts.

Nephroureterectomy. This is the operation of choice for unilateral renal tuberculosis caused by resistant organisms. Some surgeons carry it out for widespread unilateral tuberculosis with extensive cavitation even if the organisms are sensitive, because they feel that antitubercular drugs may not achieve a high enough concentration in a grossly disorganized kidney with an impaired blood supply.

Cavernotomy. A sealed-off lesion may form in a kidney if the neck of a calyx becomes stenosed by fibrosis. The operation of cavernotomy consists of excising the outer shell of the abscess and curetting the inside.

Ureter. Although tuberculosis may involve the whole ureter, it has a predilection for the lower third, which is involved first by infiltration with tuberculous follicles and later by fibrosis. A stricture may form with dilatation of the ureter and pelvis above it. The stricture may be dilated by passing bougies from below through a cystoscope or from above by open operation. Alternatively the ureter can be divided above the stricture and the proximal end reimplanted into the bladder.

Bladder. The use of cortico-steroids together with anti-tuberculous chemotherapy has reduced the incidence of the contracted bladder, which results from fibrosis. A contracted bladder can be treated by an ileo- or colo-cystoplasty, which enlarges the capacity of the bladder. Alternatively urine may be diverted into the colon or on to the skin.

NON-INFECTIVE DISORDERS OF THE BLADDER

Interstitial cystitis or Hunner's ulcer. This is a disease of unknown aetiology and primarily affects the submucosa of the bladder, which is infiltrated with plasma cells and lymphocytes. Ulcers appear on the mucosa and are typically stellate and situated in the vault of the bladder. It affects middle-aged women. Severe supra-pubic pain is experienced and relieved by micturition. The bladder capacity is reduced and frequency of micturition is much increased. The urine is sterile and contains no abnormal constituents. Antibiotics have no effect. Steroids often relieve symptoms and this fact, together with the histological appearance, have led many to suggest that the disease is an auto-immune one. Dilatation of the bladder invariably relieves symptoms for up to 6 months and is often repeated at regular intervals. In the most severe cases, operation may be required. The alternatives are urinary diversion or excision of the vault of the bladder and colo- or ileo-cystoplasty.

Phosphate encrusted cystitis. This is characterized by the deposition of phosphate or other inorganic salts on the chronically inflamed bladder wall, usually at the site of an ulcer or granulation tissue. It is most often seen when the infecting organism is *Proteus vulgaris* which splits urea and produces a strongly alkaline urine in which urinary salts are precipitated. At cystoscopy phosphatic deposits obscure the underlying mucosa, and one must be very cautious about attributing the changes to infection because phosphates can precipitate on the surface of squamous cell carcinomas.

Cystitis cystica. This is glandular metaplasia of the transitional epithelium of the bladder. Small glands form in the epithelium and project on the mucosal surface of the bladder, usually its base, as multiple tiny nodules. Sometimes the glands coalesce and form large, polypoid masses which project into the bladder and look like tumours.

Squamous carcinoma of the bladder. This often causes increased frequency of micturition, urgency and dysuria, with little, if any, haematuria. Even at cystoscopy the diagnosis can be extremely difficult because these tumours are ulcers and fissures rather than proliferative lesions and are often covered by phosphatic encrustations. The urine is usually sterile but secondary infections occur.

Bladder neck or urethral syndrome. Some 50 per cent of women who complain of persistent or intermittent frequency, dysuria and urgency have no infection and no discoverable abnormality on full pelvic and urological examination. Some respond to urethral dilatation, to antibiotics, to antispasmodics, to analgesics or to diathermy of the bladder neck. The aetiology of this syndrome is often obscure, but in many patients there is marked psychological overlay.

Many patients and some doctors, who should know better, assume that increased frequency of micturition, dysuria and urgency mean cystitis, and even persevere in this belief if the urine is sterile. These symptoms only indicate that bladder function is disturbed and the patient must be examined properly in order to find out why. Many lesions other than infection can cause symptoms of chronic cystitis, and even if the cause is infection, there must be some predisposing abnormality, like obstruction, fistula, stone or foreign body. In males, infections of

142

the prostate can cause symptoms similar to, and sometimes indistinguishable from, those of acute or chronic cystitis (p. 200).

BILHARZIA (SCHISTOSOMIASIS)

Schistosomiasis is caused by any one of the three species of parasitic worm, which has a fresh water snail as its intermediate host. *Schistosoma mansoni* and *S. japonicum* have a predilection for the gastro-intestinal tract, *S. haematobium* for the urinary tract. The adult *S. haematobium* lays its eggs in small blood vessels in the wall of the bladder or, less often, in the wall of the ureter or renal pelvis. The spiked ova penetrate the lining of the urinary tract and enter the urine. As they pass through the urinary tract they damage its epithelium and produce ulcers which bleed. Later, papillary growths of granulation tissue and stones form and secondary infection and fibrosis are common. If the ureters are involved, strictures form and hydro- and even pyo-nephrosis occurs. The irritation of the bladder may cause metaplasia and later squamous carcinoma.

Prophylaxis and treatment

To prevent schistosomiasis the snails which act as intermediate hosts for the parasite must be controlled or destroyed. This has not proved easy, and the infestation remains a scourge in many tropical countries. Intravenous administration of trivalent antimony salts has been used successfully since 1917, but its side effects include exfoliative dermatitis. Niridazole (Ambilhar) is an effective oral agent which has fewer side effects than antimony, but produces neurological and psychiatric disturbances in some patients.

FURTHER READING

Black, D. A. K. (1967). *Renal Disease,* 2nd ed. Oxford: Blackwell.
O'Grady, F. & Brumfitt, W. (1968). *Urinary Tract Infection.* London: Oxford University Press.
Riches, Sir Eric (1970). *Modern Trends in Urology* – 3, pp. 3–60. London: Butterworths.
Scott, J. (1968). In *Paediatric Urology,* pp. 175–195. Ed. Williams, D. I. London: Butterworths.

Chapter 9

STONES IN THE URINARY TRACT

Although stones are found in the kidney, the ureter, the bladder and the urethra, they are formed only in the kidney and the bladder. Renal stones usually lie free in the pelvis or calyces, but may have a tenuous attachment to the epithelium. They are to be distinguished from nephrocalcinosis, which is calcification in the parenchyma of the kidney.

All urinary calculi consist of crystalloids laid down on an organic matrix. The matrix is a mucoprotein united by strong chemical bonds with a sulphated mucopolysaccharide and comprises about 2.5 per cent of the calculus. In 90 per cent of calculi the crystalloids contain calcium either as calcium oxalate with or without a small amount of calcium phosphate, or as a mixture of calcium phosphate and magnesium ammonium phosphate. In the 10 per cent of calculi that do not contain calcium, the main crystalloid is either uric acid or cystine.

Cystine stones and most calcium oxalate stones form in a calyx, usually a lower one. Calcium phosphate and uric acid stones may form not only in a calyx, but also in the renal pelvis or in the bladder.

AETIOLOGY

The following predispose to stone formation in the urinary tract:

Metabolic abnormalities (Table 6).

Urinary tract infections.

Foreign bodies in the urinary tract.

Obstruction and stasis in the urinary tract.

Geographical factors.

All patients with stones should be investigated in the hope of identifying a predisposing cause which can be found in nearly all patients with bladder stones, but in less than 20 per cent of those with renal or ureteric stones.

144

Metabolic Causes

Table 6 Metabolic causes of urinary calculi

Calcium Stones

Hypercalciuria

Hyperparathyroidism
Vitamin D intoxication
Sarcoidosis
Milk alkali syndrome
Renal tubular acidosis
Immobilization
Cushing's syndrome
Idiopathic hypercalciuria

Alkaline urine
Oxaluria

Uric Acid Stones

Uricosuria

Primary gout
Uricosuric drugs
Secondary gout

Cystine Stones

Cystinuria

Cystinuria
Cystinosis

Xanthine Stones
Xanthinuria (excessively rare)

Calcium Stones

The metabolic disorders that predispose to the formation of calcium-containing stones are: (1) hypercalciuria, which is the excretion in the urine of excessive amounts of calcium; (2) the excretion of an alkaline urine: calcium salts are relatively insoluble in alkaline media; (3) hyperoxaluria, which is the excretion in the urine of excessive amounts of oxalate: calcium oxalate is very insoluble.

Many patients with calcium-containing stones or nephrocalcinosis or both have hypercalciuria, which must be considered an aetiological factor because it seldom occurs in people who do not form stones. On a normal ward diet the amount of calcium excreted in the urine is considered excessive if it exceeds 300 mg per 24 hours in the male or 250 mg per 24 hours in the female.

Although hypercalcaemia (a raised serum calcium) causes hypercalciuria because more calcium than usual is filtered at the glomeruli, hypercalciuria occurs more often in the presence of a normal serum calcium. Hypercalcaemia also causes an increased output of hydrogen ions by both the kidneys and the stomach, and therefore is associated with an acid urine. Because calcium salts are more soluble in acid than in alkaline media, some patients with hypercalcaemia and hypercalciuria do not form stones.

Hypercalcaemia involves the kidney not only by predisposing to stone formation but also by causing nephrocalcinosis. Calcium is deposited in the tubular cells especially of the distal tubules and collecting ducts, and causes not only distal tubular dysfunction with renal diabetes insipidus and renal tubular acidosis but also, eventually, a fall in glomerular filtration rate (Chap. 4). As the glomerular filtration rate falls, less calcium is excreted in the urine because less is filtered. The calcium deposits can often be seen in plain X-rays of the kidneys and have to be distinguished from such other causes of nephrocalcinosis as infection, and medullary sponge kidney.

Primary hyperparathyroidism

In this disease, which is the commonest cause of hypercalcaemia, the parathyroid glands are hypertrophied or contain one or more adenomata and produce excessive quantities of parathormone. Parathormone reduces the reabsorption of phosphate by the renal tubules, mobilizes calcium from bone and increases the absorption of calcium from the gut. In primary hyperparathyroidism, the serum calcium level is raised, the serum phosphate level is low, and excessive quantities of calcium and phosphate are excreted in the urine. However, not so much calcium is excreted as might be expected from its serum level and there seems to be an increased reabsorption of calcium by the renal tubules.

Clinical features

Because parathyroid tumours are small and soft they can rarely be seen or palpated in the neck.

Renal involvement is the commonest manifestation of hyperparathyroidism and may take the form of recurrent renal calculi or of nephrocalcinosis. The first cause renal colic and sometimes haematuria, infection and anuria; the second polyuria, polydipsia and later renal failure.

Bony changes (osteitis fibrosa cystica) are rare in primary hyperparathyroidism but common in the secondary hyperparathyroidism of some renal diseases and malabsorption syndromes. Decalcification and cyst formation occur and cause swelling, pain and sometimes pathological fractures. The serum alkaline phosphatase is raised if there is bone involvement.

Gastro-intestinal symptoms, such as nausea, vomiting, anorexia, constipation and dysphagia frequently occur. Some patients develop peptic ulcers because hypercalcaemia increases the production of acid by the stomach, and some complain of weakness, lassitude and tiredness because hypercalcaemia reduces nerve and muscle excitability.

Diagnosis

Although an immunological method of estimating directly the amount of parathyroid hormone in serum is being developed, it is not yet available for clinical use. The estimation of the serum calcium level is still the most important investigation for the diagnosis of hyperparathyroidism. Of the total serum calcium, 60 per cent is ionized. Of the non-ionized fraction, all but 5 per cent is bound to plasma proteins, and is not filtered at the glomeruli. If the serum protein concentration rises, the protein-bound calcium rises in proportion; if the serum protein level falls, there is a fall in protein-bound calcium. Only the ionized calcium is metabolically active, and under the control of parathyroid hormone. In a fasting patient the normal upper limit for serum calcium is 10.6 mg per cent for the total and 6.5 mg per cent for the ionized fraction. The specimen must be taken without a tourniquet, because venous stasis may give falsely high values.

The urinary excretion of calcium is increased, and does not fall to normal levels if the calcium content of the diet is reduced. The serum phosphate level is low, and the renal clearance of phosphate is high.

Although bone changes are uncommon in primary hyperparathyroidism, a skeletal survey, which must include hands, skull and teeth, should be carried out, especially if the serum alkaline phosphatase is raised.

Treatment

If the criteria of hyperparathyroidism are established, the neck must be explored. The identification of parathyroid tissue is sometimes difficult and facilities for frozen section microscopy must be available. If an adenoma cannot be identified in the neck, the mediastinum must be explored.

Vitamin D intoxication

Vitamin D increases the absorption of calcium from the gut. Excessive amounts of Vitamin D (which may be given in fortified foods to young children or in vitamin supplements to patients suffering from malabsorption) cause hypercalcaemia and hypercalciuria.

Sarcoidosis

Some patients with sarcoidosis are hypersensitive to vitamin D, and develop hypercalcaemia and hypercalciuria because a normal amount of the vitamin has an exaggerated effect.

Milk-alkali syndrome

Some patients with dyspepsia develop alkalosis, hypercalcaemia and hypercalciuria because they drink large amounts of milk, and eat large quantities of alkalis, which are often calcium salts. The urine is alkaline, which increases the tendency to stone formation because calcium salts are less soluble in alkaline than in acid media. Hypercalcaemia increases the secretion of acid by the stomach, which aggravates the dyspepsia, and increases the need for milk and alkalis.

Malignant disease involving bone

When malignant cells metastasize to bone they destroy it, releasing calcium into the circulation. If the metastases are widespread, both hypercalcaemia and hypercalciuria occur and calculi may form if the patient survives long enough.

In myeloma two kinds of hypercalcaemia may occur, firstly the increase in the ionized fraction of calcium which results from widespread bone destruction and leads to hypercalciuria, and secondly an increase in the plasma-bound fraction, which is associated with the high concentration of abnormal serum proteins and which does not cause hypercalciuria.

Immobilization

With immobilization or the prolonged weightlessness of space travel, bone mass decreases because bones are no longer subjected to the normal stresses of muscular activity and weight-bearing. Large quantities of calcium are released into the blood stream and excreted in the urine.

Immobilization also causes stasis of urine, especially in the lower calyces of the kidney, which increases the risk of stone formation.

Cushing's syndrome: cortico-steroid therapy

Large amounts of adrenal steroids break down protein including the protein matrix of bone. The loss of matrix releases calcium which is excreted in the urine. Renal calculi may therefore occur in Cushing's syndrome, whether this results from adrenal overactivity or from the therapeutic administration of steroids.

Idiopathic hypercalciuria

Idiopathic hypercalciuria is the commonest cause of hypercalciuria and therefore of urinary calculi. It has been attributed to a specific tubular defect in calcium reabsorption, but is not associated with any other tubular defects. On a normal diet, the amount of calcium in a 24-hour urine is normally less than 300 mg in the male and 250 mg in the female. If the calcium content of the diet is reduced to about 150 mg, the urinary calcium gradually decreases and equals the intake within 3 or 4 days. Patients with idiopathic hypercalciuria have a normal serum calcium but excrete more than 300 mg of calcium each 24 hours, and if the calcium content of their diet is reduced, they excrete substantially more than their intake for several weeks. Most patients with idiopathic hypercalciuria are healthy, apart from their increased liability to stone formation.

Renal tubular acidosis

In this condition, the blood is relatively acid, and the urine relatively alkaline because the kidneys are unable to produce an acid urine. Protein-bound calcium dissociates in acid media and because the amount of ionized calcium in the blood increases, hypercalciuria occurs. The urine is alkaline, and as calcium salts precipitate in alkaline media, there is a marked tendency to stone formation.

149

Oxaluria

Calcium oxalate stones are often associated with hypercalciuria, but rarely with hyperoxaluria. The normal urinary excretion of oxalate is 10 to 45 mg per day, and in adults hyperoxaluria is extremely rare. Some infants, however, suffer an inborn error of glycine metabolism and excrete up to 400 mg of oxalate per day, which causes multiple bilateral renal calculi and deposits of calcium oxalate crystals in many sites throughout the body.

Uric Acid Stones

Uric acid stones, unlike calcium stones, are no more radio-opaque than soft tissues, and therefore are not visible on plain X-rays.

They form in some patients with primary or secondary gout if the production of uric acid in the body and therefore its urinary excretion are increased.

Secondary gout occurs in diseases such as leukaemia, polycythaemia and haemolytic anaemias when cell turnover is rapid, and large amounts of nucleic acids, which are excreted as uric acid, are released. X-rays or cytotoxic drugs cause a massive destruction of immature cells in leukaemia or polycythaemia and serum uric acid levels may increase tenfold.

Some patients with raised serum uric acid levels excrete a normal amount of uric acid and show no tendency to form stones. However, if they are given uricosuric drugs uric acid excretion increases and stones may form.

Some patients with normal serum and urinary uric acid levels form uric acid stones because they excrete a strongly acid urine and uric acid is less soluble in acid than in alkaline media.

Cystine Stones

A 24-hour collection of urine normally contains less than 0.5 mg of the amino acid cystine. In two conditions, cystinuria and cystinosis, it contains excessive amounts of up to 0.5 g or even 1.0 g. Cystine is relatively insoluble, more so in acid than in alkaline urine, and may precipitate and form stones. Cystine stones are only slightly more radio-opaque than soft tissues, and therefore are not usually visible on plain X-rays.

Cystinuria. Cystinuria is an inborn defect in the tubular reabsorption of four amino acids, cystine, lysine, ornithine and arginine, but only cystine is insoluble enough to form stones. It is inherited as an autosomal recessive and only homozygotes excrete enough cystine to form stones. In some families heterozygotes have minor defects of amino acid reabsorption, in others no abnormality can be detected.

Cystinosis. Cystinosis is also an inborn error of metabolism of recessive nature. It is more complex than cystinuria, and causes not only the excretion of excessive quantities of cystine, but also the Fanconi syndrome (Chap. 4).

Patients with the Fanconi syndrome are unable to concentrate and acidify urine and pass a dilute alkaline urine in which cystine is relatively soluble. The formation of cystine stones is therefore less of a problem than in cystinuria, but cystine is often deposited in numerous other sites throughout the body. Patients with the Fanconi syndrome have renal tubular acidosis and may form calcium stones, or develop nephrocalcinosis.

Xanthine Stones

Xanthinuria is a rare disease in which there are excessive quantities of xanthine and hypoxanthine, the precursors of uric acid in urine. It is caused by a defect in the enzyme xanthine oxidase, which may be inherited or may follow the treatment of gout with Allopurinol. Xanthine is more soluble than uric acid, and xanthine stones are excessively rare.

Infection

Infection predisposes to stone formation but it is often hard to determine whether the stone or the infection came first.

Urea-splitting organisms, such as proteus, make the urine alkaline by producing ammonia, and thus tend to promote the formation of calcium phosphate stones. Any infection increases the amount of organic debris in the urine, and such debris may act as a nucleus for stone formation.

Foreign Bodies

Foreign bodies in the urinary tract, such as non-absorbable

151

sutures or nephrostomy tubes, predispose to the formation of stones, firstly by providing a nidus for calcium phosphate deposition and secondly by predisposing to infection.

Obstruction and Stasis

Epithelial cells and other organic debris shed into the urinary tract are normally carried away by the free flow of urine. If there is obstruction or stasis they may be retained and act as nuclei for stone formation. Obstruction and stasis also predispose to infection.

Geographical Factors

The incidence of urinary stones varies considerably from one country to another. This has been attributed to variations in diet, the hardness of drinking water, climate, geological and genetic factors. In hot countries, much water is lost from the skin by sweating and the urine is very concentrated. In some countries bilharziasis is endemic and the spiked ova of the worm that causes it not only cause infection but also act as nuclei for stone formation.

The mystery is perhaps not why some people form stones, but why the rest of us do not. In any reasonably concentrated urine, calcium salts are present in supersaturated solution, and why they do not precipitate and form stones in the entire population is by no means clear. Some believe that certain constituents of urine like citrates and urinary mucopolysaccharides hold calcium in solution, and that stones form if their excretion is defective. Much experimental work is being done along these lines, but at the time of writing, it remains inconclusive.

CLINICAL FEATURES

Renal and Ureteric Calculi

Renal calculi may lie in a calyx (usually a lower one) or in the renal pelvis. They may be small or large, single or multiple. Large stones form a cast of the renal pelvis and calyces, and because of their shape are called staghorn calculi (Fig. 32).

Ureteric calculi are formed in the kidney and pass down into

152

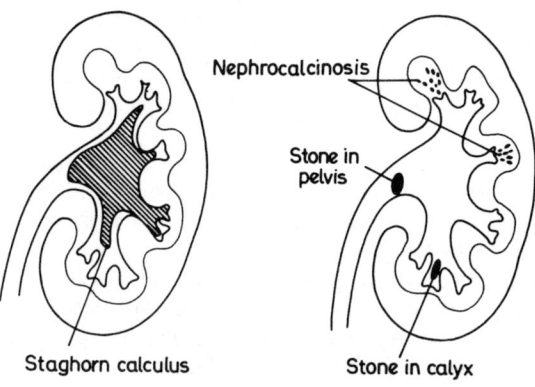

Nephrocalcinosis

Stone in pelvis

Staghorn calculus

Stone in calyx

Fig. 32.

the ureter. They may increase in size if they remain in the ureter for any length of time. Very small stones may pass on into the bladder without causing symptoms, but most impact and produce a greater or lesser degree of obstruction.

The symptoms of renal and ureteric calculi depend on the degree of obstruction to the flow of urine, on the extent of mucosal irritation, and on whether or not there is accompanying infection.

Pain. Renal or ureteric colic occurs if the stone impacts and causes sudden and severe obstruction. If the obstruction is incomplete or occurs gradually, pain is much less severe and may be aggravated by drinking. Low grade inflammatory changes may develop in perinephric or periureteric tissues if the stone remains in one place for some time, and cause pain. Renal and ureteric colic are associated with nausea, sweating and restlessness. The site of the pain and the extent of its radiation depend upon the level of obstruction. If the stone is at the pelvi-ureteric junction, pain may be confined to the loin, if it is in the ureter, pain may begin in the loin, but radiates to iliac fossa, groin, external genitalia or even thigh.

Haematuria. Stones are often irregular and jagged and may abrade the mucosa of the renal tract, causing haematuria.

Infection. Stones predispose to infection not only by causing obstruction but also by abrading the mucosa of the renal tract. Both acute and chronic pyelonephritis may occur. Acute infection in an obstructed kidney may be very severe, causing pain, high

153

fever, rigors, and sometimes septicaemia, and may progress to pyonephrosis if the obstruction is not relieved.

Acute renal failure. Acute renal failure occurs if both ureters or the ureter of a solitary kidney are completely obstructed by stone.

Metaplasia. Prolonged irritation or infection may produce metaplasia, which is a change in cell type from transitional epithelium to squamous epithelium. Although this is symptomless, it may progress to malignant change.

Chronic renal failure. Stones in both kidneys or in a solitary kidney together with the infection and obstruction associated with them may severely damage the parenchyma of the kidney and lead to chronic, irreversible renal failure.

Bladder symptoms. Bladder symptoms may result from cystitis secondary to the upper urinary tract infection caused by stone. If a calculus impacts in the intramural part of the ureter, the ureteric orifice becomes oedematous and protrudes into and irritates the bladder, causing frequency of micturition and penile pain.

Bladder Stones

Primary bladder stones, that is stones which form in normal non-infected bladders, are common in some eastern countries and are attributed to dietary factors. In this country all bladder stones are secondary to local disorders such as obstruction, infection and foreign bodies, the symptoms of which may overshadow those caused by the stone. Stones in the bladder can cause haematuria, recurrent or chronic cystitis, obstruction and strangury. Strangury is a severe supra-pubic or urethral pain that radiates to the tip of the penis occurring during or immediately after micturition, and associated with an urgent desire to pass urine, even though the bladder is empty. Only a few drops of fresh blood may be passed if micturition is attempted.

Diagnosis of Urinary Stones

The history and clinical examination may suggest that there are stones in the urinary tract, but only X-ray examinations can demonstrate them. All calcium-containing stones are more opaque than soft tissue, and will be visible in straight X-rays, provided that they are not too small and do not overlie calcified structures like ribs, transverse processes or the sacrum. Uric acid stones are always and cystine stones are usually no more radio-opaque than soft tissues and therefore cannot be seen in plain X-rays. If they lie in the kidneys or ureters they can, however, be demonstrated as filling defects in intravenous or retrograde pyelograms; if they lie in the bladder, they can be seen at cystoscopy.

MANAGEMENT

The management of patients suffering from urinary calculus can be discussed under certain headings.

Urgent or Acute Symptoms

Renal or ureteric colic. Renal colic can be relieved by strong analgesics or smooth muscle relaxants. When the stone impacts there is sudden severe obstruction and therefore pain. After a time, some urine manages to find its way past the stone and pain is relieved. A second attack of pain especially if it is at a lower level means that the stone has moved and impacted at a lower level in the ureter.

Severe infection. Acute infection in an obstructed kidney can be very severe and cause high fevers and rigors with an enlarged palpable kidney and sometimes septicaemia, although the urine may contain neither pus nor organisms. Relief of the obstruction may be imperative.

Acute renal failure. If the patient has acute renal failure, relief of the obstruction is imperative.

Urinary retention. Urinary retention caused by a stone that impacts in the bladder neck can be relieved by catheterization. Retention caused by a stone in the urethra can usually be relieved only by removal of the stone.

Investigation to Find out the Cause of the Stones

Although detailed biochemical tests should probably be

155

carried out in all patients with calculi, only in those patients with recurrent, bilateral or multiple stones, with non-opaque stones, with a family history of stone, with stones and nephrocalcinosis, and with stones associated with symptoms that suggest bone disease or duodenal ulcer or with obstruction or infection and with bladder stones are these investigations at all likely to reveal the cause.

The estimation of calcium, phosphate, oxalate, uric acid and cystine in three 24-hour specimens of urine will demonstrate hypercalciuria, hyperoxaluria, uricosuria or cystinuria. The estimation of calcium, phosphate, uric acid, plasma proteins, alkaline phosphatase in the blood will demonstrate hypercalcaemia, hyperuricaemia and the possibility of bone disease. The calcium must be assessed in fasting blood on, at the very least, three separate occasions. X-rays of the skeleton or at least of the skull, teeth and hands should be made, and three or more midstream specimens of urine should be cultured. A urological examination may be required to exclude stasis, obstruction or foreign bodies.

In all patients suffering from bladder stones, the cause should be apparent, and is usually infection, obstruction or a foreign body. Metabolic disorders do not cause bladder calculi.

In patients with renal or ureteric stones idiopathic hypercalciuria is found in 50 per cent; other causes of hypercalciuria, e.g. hyperparathyroidism, cystinuria or gout, are found in 10 per cent. In 40 per cent no defect other than the stones is found.

Treatment of Stones

Kidney

Small stones may pass, and can be observed unless they are causing symptoms. Larger stones should be removed.

Of the various solutions suggested for dissolving stones none is effective for use in kidney or ureter, although some soft stones like those made up of cystine can be reduced in size by diuresis. If the stone is large, or if it fails to pass after a reasonable time, one of the following operations is carried out.

Pyelolithotomy. This is removal of a stone through an incision in the pelvis of the kidney. It is used mostly for stones in the pelvis and for some in the calyces.

Nephrolithotomy. This is the removal of a stone from a calyx of the kidney by means of an incision through the parenchyma of the kidney.

Partial nephrectomy. This is the removal of a stone in a calyx together with the calyx and associated parenchyma. It is a good operation when there is a stone or stones in one calyx.

Nephrectomy. Both the stone and the whole kidney are sometimes removed if the stone is large or if there are many stones, provided that the other kidney is normal.

If both kidneys contain stones the appropriate operation should be carried out on each, the best kidney being done first and the other some weeks later. If each kidney contains a staghorn stone, operation should be considered only if the patient has severe pain, severe infection or severe bleeding, and then an attempt should be made to remove the stones.

Ureter

Ninety per cent of ureteric stones pass spontaneously and the patient should be treated conservatively, but surgical intervention is urgent if there is severe infection or acute renal failure and desirable soon if there are repeated attacks of pain with no sign of the stone moving, infection, progressive hydronephrosis, or if the stone seems too large to pass.

If intervention is necessary an attempt can be made to remove the stone by endoscopic means if it is less than 1 cm in diameter and lies in the lower third of the ureter. The alternative is open operation (uretero-lithotomy).

Bladder

Most stones in the bladder are secondary to obstruction at the bladder neck or in the urethra, or develop in diverticula. It is essential that the obstruction is treated as well as the stone. Most obstructive lesions are treated by open operation, and it is a simple matter to remove the stone at the same time. If, however, it is decided to remove the stone but not to do anything more to the lower urinary tract (as is often the case with neurological disturbances of the bladder or with stones that form after a prolonged period of catheter drainage), the stone can either be crushed with a lithotrite and the fragments washed out of the bladder or it can be removed by open operation.

Urethra

Stones that enter the urethra can usually pass through with

little difficulty, but some impact either at the external meatus (the narrowest part of the urethra) or proximal to a urethral stricture. Stones impacted at the external meatus can easily be removed if the meatus is incised and enlarged (meatotomy). Stones impacted more proximally in the urethra can either be pushed back into the bladder with a urethral bougie and then crushed with a lithotrite, or be removed through a small incision in the skin and urethra.

Infection

Infection that persists after the stone is removed must be energetically treated with antibiotics.

Chronic Renal Failure

The treatment of chronic renal failure is discussed in Chapters 4 and 5.

Prevention of Recurrent Stones

To prevent the recurrence of stones is as important as treating the ones already present. Bladder stones should not recur after the obstruction, infection or foreign body that caused them is eradicated, but the prevention of renal and ureteric calculi can be much more difficult. Fortunately many patients with renal or ureteric stones have only one attack, and, provided that the stone is a solitary calcium one and unassociated with features that suggest a predisposing cause, they require no special treatment and are often not even subjected to the special investigations (p. 155).

Patients with recurrent or multiple stones or stones composed of uric acid or cystine must be investigated. If a predisposing cause is found and can be eradicated, no further stones should form. Unfortunately, in few such patients is a cause like hyperparathyroidism, milk alkali syndrome, hypervitaminosis D, obstruction or foreign body, found.

Nevertheless even in patients in whom a predisposing cause is either not found or cannot be treated, there are some measures which can be taken to discourage stone formation. They should drink copiously in order to maintain a rapid flow of dilute urine for the whole 24 hours. Urine is usually very concentrated during the night regardless of the fluid intake during the day and the patient must drink at least a pint of fluid before going to bed and again when he wakes up to pass urine. Slight insomnia is a small price to pay for the prevention of stones. Sodium bicarbonate alkalinizes the urine and should be given to patients with uric acid and cystine stones, both of which are more soluble in alkaline than in acid media. Allopurinol reduces the production of uric acid and can be given to patients with uric acid stones. Penicillamine, a chelating agent, increases the solubility of cystine and can be given to patients with cystine stones.

In some patients with idiopathic hypercalciuria, stones recur despite a high fluid intake. They can be advised to take a diet which is low in calcium and oxalate content and avoid foods like spinach and rhubarb, which are rich in oxalate, reduce their intake of milk and cheese, which are rich in calcium, and drink distilled instead of tap water if they live in a hard water area. However, even this diet may not reduce the urinary excretion of calcium. Some diuretics, including bendrofluazide, reduce the urinary excretion of calcium and can be given to selected patients.

FURTHER READING

Stewart, H. H. (1965). In *Clinical Surgery,* Vol. 6. Ed. Fergusson, J. D. London: Butterworths.
Strauss, M. B. & Welt, L. G. (1963). *Diseases of the Kidney.* London: Churchill.
Winsbury-White, H. P. (1961). *Textbook of Genito-Urinary Surgery,* 2nd ed., pp. 293–335. Edinburgh: Livingstone.

Chapter 10

TUMOURS OF THE KIDNEY, URETER AND BLADDER

TUMOURS OF THE KIDNEY

Tumours can develop from any component of the renal parenchyma or from the epithelium of the calyces and pelvis. They may also develop from the connective, vascular and nerve tissues of the capsule, the perinephric tissues or the hilum of the kidney.

Tumours of the Renal Parenchyma

Pathology

The kidneys are derived from the mesoderm of the intermediate cell mass, which is totipotent and which differentiates into the epithelial, connective, vascular, fatty and smooth muscular tissues of the adult kidney. Although any of these tissues may undergo neoplastic change only the commoner tumours (Table 7) are considered here.

Table 7 The commoner tumours of the renal parenchyma

> Adenoma
> Other benign tumours
> Carcinoma of the kidney
> Embryomas
> Sarcomas
> Reticuloses
> Metastatic tumours

Adenoma

An adenoma is a benign tumour and composed of large, clear or small granular epithelial cells which form tubular, alveolar or more commonly papillary patterns. They are circumscribed, though not truly encapsulated and usually less than 1 cm in

160

diameter. They may be yellow, grey or red in colour and most are firm in consistence but some are soft or cystic. They are usually found incidentally at post-mortem examination, often in the fibrous parts of ischaemic or chronically infected kidneys, and rarely if ever cause symptoms.

Other benign tumours

Of the other benign tumours lipomas, fibromas, leiomyomas, rhabdomyomas and neurofibromas are all small and detected at post-mortem examination as small nodules indistinguishable from one another except by microscopic examination. They can be grouped together and called 'capsulomata'. The hamartoma and the haemangioma, however, are two benign tumours which deserve special mention.

Hamartoma. Some benign tumours consist of two or more cell types and can be called angiomyolipomas, angioleiomyomas, etc., after the type of cells found in them. Such tumours were first described by Albrecht in 1904, who defined them as abnormal mixtures of normal tissue elements forming tumour-like masses, and who called them 'hamartomas'. Although some hamartomas are large and bleed and necrose like carcinomas, most are small and cause no symptoms.

Haemangioma. Haemangiomas may be found anywhere in the kidney but usually lie in the submucosa of the papillae, calyces or pelvis, and cause thickening or ulceration of the overlying epithelium. They consist of dilated blood spaces lined by flattened endothelial cells and filled with blood clots. They may cause haematuria, but are usually too small to show up as filling defects in pyelograms, and have too small a blood flow to reveal themselves in angiograms.

Carcinoma of the kidney

Von Grawitz called this tumour 'hypernephroma' because he mistakenly thought it developed from adrenal rests, which are small yellow nodules of ectopic adrenal tissue frequently found in the kidneys. It is now known that carcinomas of the kidney arise from the nephron, probably from the cells of the tubule. Like other tumours they may take many forms but to classify them as adenocarcinoma, papillary-carcinoma, etc., is difficult and unhelpful because many are pleomorphic. Carcinomas of the kidney have a pseudo-capsule of compressed renal tissue and are divided into compartments by fine trabeculae. They can be solid, but part and sometimes all of the tumour is usually haemorrhagic or necrotic. Necrotic tissue eventually liquefies and forms cysts, which may be large, filled with dirty brown fluid. Solid tumours are yellow but haemorrhage and necrosis give them a variegated appearance of orange, yellow, red and brown colours. The tumours consist of large clear or small granular cells, which form solid, glandular, tubular or papillary patterns but both the appearance and the arrangement of the cells can vary markedly within a single tumour. The stromal tissue between these cells contains many dilated veins and may be partially calcified.

Carcinoma of the kidney spreads (a) by direct growth into the perinephric tissues and adjacent viscera, (b) by the blood stream to the lungs, bone, skin and almost any other part of the body, (c) by the lymphatics to the regional lymph nodes along the aorta. Tumour cells may grow along the renal vein into and up the inferior vena cava, and one of the first of these tumours to be described had extended along the inferior vena cava as far as the right atrium of the heart. Renal carcinoma has an unusual predilection for spreading by the blood stream rather than by the lymphatics. Sometimes a blood-borne metastasis is solitary and many patients have been cured by removal of both the primary tumour and a solitary metastasis. About 1 per cent of carcinomas of the kidney produce excessive quantities of the hormone erythropoietin and cause polycythaemia.

Nephroblastoma (embryoma or Wilms' tumour)

Nephroblastomas develop from immature or embryonic cells of the mesoderm of the intermediate cell mass before they differentiate into renal parenchyma. Mesoderm is totipotent and can form vascular, tubular, muscular, cartilaginous, adipose and fibroblastic tissues. Nephroblastomas account for 20 per cent of malignant tumours in childhood and are found twice as often in boys as in girls. They all appear before the age of 7 years and have been found in new-born and premature infants and even in the foetus. The tumour is highly malignant and grows rapidly, and is usually larger than the kidney itself when first discovered.

The tumour is divided into compartments by fibrous septa, but soon acquires an irregular, variegated appearance from

162

necrosis and haemorrhage. When small it may appear encapsulated, but soon infiltrates and destroys the renal parenchyma and the perinephric tissues and displaces and infiltrates adjacent organs. Later it spreads by the blood stream to the lungs. The small spindle-shaped, elongated mesodermal cells of the tumour may remain undifferentiated or may differentiate into epithelial, connective, cartilaginous, bony, fatty, or mucous cells or smooth and striated muscle fibres. The cells form solid sheets of tissue, but the epithelial ones may differentiate into tubules and glomeruli which are usually primitive but which may be almost as well differentiated as normal ones.

Sarcomas

Sarcomas can arise from connective tissue in the capsule of the kidney, in the parenchyma or in the hilum, and may be fibrosarcomas, liposarcomas, leiomyosarcomas or mixtures of all three. They can be differentiated or anaplastic, but all are malignant, and both macroscopically and microscopically they resemble sarcoma elsewhere in the body. They spread by the blood stream to the lungs and clinically are usually indistinguishable from carcinomas.

Reticulosis

Of the many reticuloses, lymphosarcoma and leukaemia are the two most likely to involve the kidney.

Lymphosarcoma may involve one or both kidneys as either small discrete nodules, or a diffuse infiltration, or large bulky tumour-like masses, and on cut section have the same grey, firm, rubbery appearance in the kidney as elsewhere.

Leukaemias may involve one or both kidneys as multiple small nodules which may be numerous and dense enough to enlarge, sometimes considerably, the size of the kidneys.

Metastatic tumours

Bronchogenic carcinoma is the tumour that most commonly metastasizes to the kidney, and Gallatzie and Payne found metastases in the kidney in 17.5 per cent of a series of patients who had died from that disease. Renal metastases are usually found after the primary tumour has been detected or treated, or at post-mortem examination, and the kidney is only one of several organs affected.

163

Clinical Features

Haematuria. About 30 per cent of patients with carcinoma and sarcoma, but few patients with nephroblastoma complain of haematuria, which is often not only the first but the only symptom. Haematuria, which may be continuous or intermittent, may be so slight as to be detected only by microscopy, or so much as to exsanguinate the patient. Sometimes elongated blood clots, forming casts of a segment of ureter, are passed and cause renal colic. Haematuria occurs only when the tumour is congested or large enough to invade the pelvis or the calyces, and often indicates advanced disease, even though it is the first symptom experienced by the patient.

Swelling. The tumour is palpable on abdominal examination in about 40 per cent of patients with carcinomas and sarcomas, and in about 80 per cent of patients with nephroblastomas when they are first seen.

Pain. Pain occurs in about 30 per cent of patients with parenchymatous tumours. It may be a dull fixed renal pain, caused by stretching of the renal capsule, by traction on the renal pedicle of the enlarged heavy kidney, or by invasion of the perinephric structures, or it may be renal or ureteric colic, caused by blood or fragments of tumour passing down the ureter.

Fever. Some patients have no local signs or symptoms of tumour but complain instead of fever, malaise, vague ill-health, generalized weakness, anorexia and weight loss. As they often have a leucocytosis and a raised erythrocyte sedimentation rate, carcinoma of the kidney must be considered as a possible diagnosis when patients with 'pyrexia of unknown origin' are investigated.

Blood changes. Blood changes occur late in the disease, although many patients are anaemic if they have bled or have widespread metastases. Conversely, about 1 per cent of patients with renal carcinoma are polycythaemic because the tumour secretes erythropoietin, which regulates red cell mass.

Blood pressure. Tumours may cause hypertension if they compress the larger blood vessels of the kidney or cause polycythaemia.

Varicocele. A left varicocele develops if tumour invades the left renal vein and obliterates the entry of the left testicular vein. The right testicular vein drains into the inferior vena cava and is rarely obstructed.

164

Metastases. About 30 per cent of patients present with symptoms and signs of metastasis, rather than of the primary tumour. Metastases can be in any part of the body, but are most common, especially from sarcomas and nephroblastomas, in the lungs, bones or brain. In the lungs, metastases can be seen in X-rays as multiple, spherical, discrete opacities in the peripheral lung fields long before they cause such symptoms as cough, haemoptysis or pleuritic pain. In bones, metastases are osteolytic and cause bone pain and spontaneous fractures.

Diagnosis

The diagnosis of tumours of the renal parenchyma is suggested by a history of haematuria, pain, vague ill-health, and by the detection of an enlarged kidney, blood abnormalities, metastases or varicocele. It can usually be confirmed by intravenous or retrograde pyelography in which the tumour appears as a space-occupying lesion which distorts, displaces, elongates or destroys one or more calyces or the pelvis of the kidney (Fig. 33).

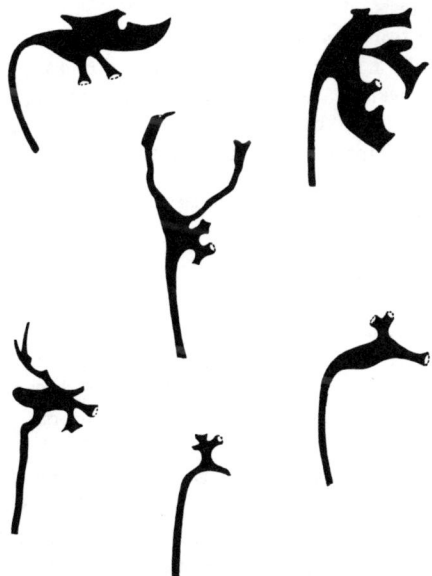

Fig. 33. Some typical appearances of the pelvi-calyceal system in pyelograms made of kidneys containing carcinoma.

Aortography or selective renal angiography may reveal a tumour by demonstrating enlargement of the renal artery, abnormal blood vessels and pooling of blood in venous sinuses, but is by no means infallible in distinguishing between tumours and a solitary cyst (the space-occupying lesion most often confused with tumour) because some tumours are relatively avascular. Examination of the urine for exfoliated cells is of little, if any, value.

Treatment

Carcinoma of the kidney. Primary carcinoma of the kidney is not very sensitive to X-rays and is best treated by nephrectomy. To excise the ureter along with the kidney is seldom necessary because the tumour rarely spreads down the ureter. The renal vein should be clamped and ligated at an early stage of the operation so that malignant cells or pieces of tumour are not disseminated into the circulation while the kidney is being mobilized. Sometimes a blood-borne metastasis is solitary and many patients have been cured by removal of both the primary tumour and the solitary metastasis.

It has been found possible to produce carcinoma of the kidney in Syrian male hamsters with relative ease. In Syrian female hamsters, however, it was found that such tumours could be produced only at times of low progesterone output such as after oophorectomy. This work suggests that some carcinomas of the kidney are hormone-dependent. Progesterone or testosterone therapy may be tried in patients who have incurable or recurrent tumours, but the response is usually disappointing. Other chemotherapeutic agents are of little or no value.

Sarcoma. Sarcomas present with similar features to carcinomas and therefore are unlikely to be diagnosed until nephrectomy has been carried out. Local or distant recurrences, however, are more sensitive to X-ray therapy than those of carcinoma.

Nephroblastoma. X-ray therapy will often shrink these tumours to a remarkable extent, but rarely cures them and should be followed by nephrectomy. Many surgeons use chemotherapeutic agents, especially actinomycin-D, in addition to X-ray therapy and surgery.

TUMOURS OF RENAL PELVIS, URETER AND BLADDER

Pathology

The calyces, the pelves, the ureters and the bladder are lined by transitional cell epithelium, which Melicow called 'urothelium', and most tumours that arise from these structures are formed from transitional cells. However, squamous or glandular carcinoma can occur if neoplastic change takes place in an area of metaplasia.

A transitional cell tumour begins as a tiny focus of abnormal cell proliferation upon or within the epithelium. Later it appears on the mucosal surface as a proliferative lesion, which may have a thin pedicle and thin delicate villi each consisting of a core of stromal tissue and blood vessels covered by one or more layers of transitional epithelial cells, or which may be sessile and solid, consisting of layers of epithelial cells without pedicle or villi. The cells of the tumour may closely resemble those of normal transitional epithelium but variations in size, shape and staining qualities, and varying degrees of hyperchromatism, polynucleosis and anaplasia are often found. Although some transitional cell tumours confine themselves to the mucosa, others penetrate the basement membrane, and invade the underlying muscle and later the structures outside the renal pelvis, ureter or bladder.

Tumours which have a thin pedicle and thin delicate villi, which are covered by normal transitional cells, and which do not penetrate the basement membranes can be called 'papillomas'. All other tumours are carcinomas and can be classified by their appearance as papillary or solid, pedunculated or sessile, by their histology as differentiated or anaplastic, and by their depth of infiltration as mucosal, muscular, or peripelvic, periureteric or perivesical. There is, however, often no clear distinction either clinically or pathologically between papillomas and carcinomas because histological appearances may vary so much from one part of the tumour to another, and because even papillomas tend to recur.

Transitional cell tumours are often multiple and if one is found, there may well be others elsewhere in the urinary tract. Some believe that the development of even one small transitional cell tumour is evidence enough that the whole of the urothelium is unstable.

167

Tumours in the renal pelvis may obstruct the pelvi-ureteric junction and cause hydronephrosis, and other effects of obstruction, like infection. Tumours in the ureter are often compressed by its narrow lumen and elongated by its peristalsis. Some but by no means all ureteric tumours cause obstruction and to demonstrate a normal renal pelvis and normal upper ureter does not exclude serious ureteric disease. Most tumours in the bladder originate on the base near the ureteric orifices, and obstruct one or even both ureters if and when they infiltrate the muscle of the bladder (Fig. 34).

If neoplastic change occurs in areas of metaplasia, glandular or squamous tumours develop. Glandular metaplasia is called pyelitis cystica, ureteritis cystica or cystitis cystica, depending on the site affected. The submucosa contains simple glands whose secretions

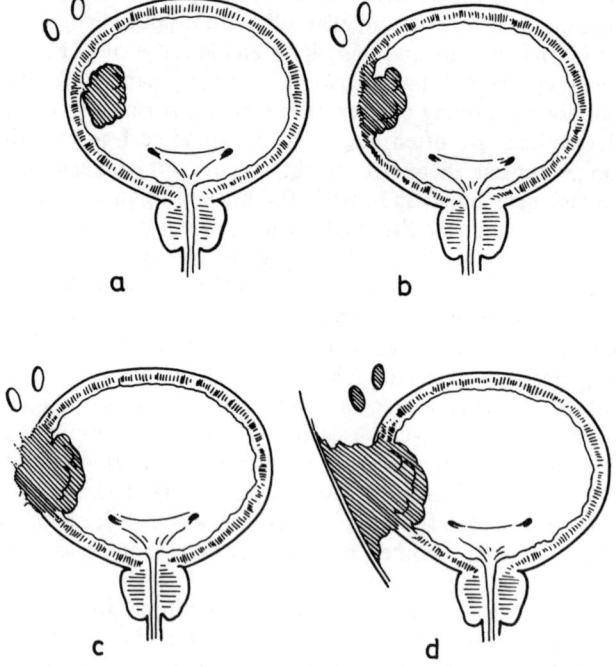

Fig. 34. Stages in progression of a carcinoma of the bladder. a. Mucosal. b. Muscular. c. Perivesical. d. Perivesical with fixation to the side wall of the pelvis and metastases in lymph nodes.

escape on to the surface or accumulate inside the gland to form small cysts, which protrude into the lumen. If they become malignant, adenocarcinoma, often of the mucoid type, develops.

Squamous metaplasia is usually a complication of chronic irritation and is therefore found in kidneys or bladders that are infected, obstructed or contain stone. It is sometimes called 'leucoplakia', but differs from leucoplakia of the mouth or tongue because it is a change in the type of epithelium rather than an over-development of existing epithelium. Glandular or squamous metaplasia determines what type of tumour develops, but neither is more liable to malignant change than normal transitional epithelium. Squamous or epidermoid carcinoma is usually an infiltrative type of growth with much fibrosis, and is often obscured by infection or encrustation.

Although most tumours of the renal pelves, ureter and bladder are primary, all three structures may be involved in tumours that spread from adjacent organs. The lower end of one or both ureters is often involved and obstructed by malignant disease of the cervix, prostate or rectum, and pyelonephritis and chronic renal failure are frequently found in the terminal stages of these diseases. Tumours of the colon, rectum and cervix may invade the bladder and form vesico-colic, vesico-rectal and vesico-vaginal fistulae respectively (p. 195).

Clinical Features of Tumours of Renal Pelvis and Ureter

Ninety-five per cent of patients with tumours in the renal pelvis and ureters present with haematuria. If a calyx or the pelvis or the ureter is obstructed by the tumour, by fragments of tumour that have broken off or even by blood clot, the patient may complain of pain or any of the other effects of obstruction.

Tumours of the renal pelvis and of the ureter appear as filling defects in intravenous or retrograde pyelograms, which may also reveal obstruction. Filling defects can also be produced by blood clot, stone and air bubbles, and considerable care must be exercised in their interpretation. The ureters are difficult to demonstrate radiologically and few intravenous pyelograms show their whole lengths. Retrograde ureterograms, obtained by injecting dye into the ureter through a ureteric catheter, are essential if ureteric tumours are suspected.

Clinical Features of Tumours of the Bladder

The bladder is by far the commonest site for tumours in the urinary tract. Malignant tumours eventually invade the muscle of the bladder and the perivesical tissues, involving and obstructing one or both ureters. Over 90 per cent of patients with bladder tumours present with painless haematuria, but squamous carcinomas, which account for 5 per cent of all bladder tumours, are often ulcers or fissures covered by phosphatic encrustations, and present not with haematuria, but with increased frequency of micturition and dysuria, and simulate chronic cystitis. Through a cystoscope, the appearance, site, number and size of the bladder tumours can be noted, and a biopsy taken. The extent to which the tumour has infiltrated the bladder and perivesical tissues can be assessed by bimanual examination. An intravenous pyelogram is mandatory. It may demonstrate the tumour as a filling defect in the bladder, it reveals ureteric obstruction, which occurs only when the tumour has infiltrated the muscle of the bladder or the perivesical tissues, and it may reveal other transitional cell tumours in the ureters or renal pelves (Table 8).

Table 8 The TNM method of expressing the stage of a bladder tumour

T = Primary Tumour (histological and bimanual examination).
　　　T1 Tumour with subepithelial infiltration only.
　　　T2 Tumour with infiltration of superficial muscle.
　　　T3 Tumour with infiltration of deep muscle.
　　　T4 Tumour fixed or invading adjacent organs.

N = Regional Lymph Nodes (can be assessed only if laparotomy is carried out).
　　　N−　Lymph nodes not involved
　　　N+　Lymph nodes involved.

M = Distant Metastases
　　　M = Metastases detected.
　　　MO = Metastases not detected.

Treatment

Tumours of renal pelvis and ureter. Tumours of the renal pelvis and ureter are treated by removing the kidney together with the entire length of the ureter. However, if the other kidney or ureter contains tumour or is otherwise abnormal, treatment may have to be limited to a local excision of the tumour.

Tumours of the bladder. Tumours that are villous and pedunculated, confined to the mucosa and composed of cells that closely resemble those of normal transitional epithelium can be destroyed by diathermy which can be applied either through a cystoscope or a resectoscope, or by open operation. Other tumours are best treated by X-ray therapy. For solitary tumours that are less than 4 cm in diameter and extend no further into the bladder than the superficial muscle, interstitial radiation using tantulum wire, radium needles or radon seeds is used. For others radiation is given from an external source like a linear accelerator or cobalt bomb. Partial cystectomy should be carried out only for tumours in the vault of the bladder, which is an uncommon site for tumours, because it is satisfactory only if the tumour can be excised together with a 2.5 cm margin all round of normal bladder. Total cystectomy is reserved for tumours which recur after or do not respond to radiotherapy and cannot be controlled by diathermy, yet still seem confined to the bladder. If cystectomy is carried out the urine must be diverted and the ureters transplanted into the colon or on to skin. Incurable tumours of the bladder often cause severe haematuria, frequency and dysuria, which may be relieved only by transplanting the ureters into the colon.

Certain chemicals, particularly B-naphthylamine and benzidine, which were used in the chemical, rubber, plastic and gas industries, are known to have carcinogenic effects on transitional epithelium and transitional cell tumours are now recognized as an occupational disease in workers who have been exposed to these chemicals. It is important to enquire carefully into the present and past occupations of all patients with tumours of the renal pelvis, ureter and bladder since they may be entitled to industrial benefits.

All patients with tumours of the bladder, no matter how simple the tumour and how effective the treatment, must be followed up at regular intervals by cystoscopy in order to recognize recurrent tumour at an early stage, when further treatment may be effective.

FURTHER READING

Riches, Sir Eric (Ed.). (1970). *Modern Trends in Urology* – 3. pp. 163–278. London: Butterworths.

Wallace, D. M. (1960). *Monographs on Neoplastic Disease,* Vol. 2. *Cancer of the Bladder.* Edinburgh: Livingstone.

Willis, R. A. (1967). *Pathology of Tumours,* 4th ed., pp. 456–485. London: Butterworths.

Chapter 11

CONGENITAL DISORDERS OF THE URINARY AND MALE GENITAL TRACTS

DEVELOPMENT OF THE KIDNEY, URETERS AND BLADDER

The kidneys, the ureters and most of the bladder and urethra develop from the mesoderm of the intermediate cell mass, which also gives rise to the male and female reproductive organs.

Three embryonic structures contribute successively to the formation of the urinary tract — the pronephros, the mesonephros and the metanephros. The metanephros is the last of the three to appear, and, in humans, persists as the adult kidney (Fig. 35).

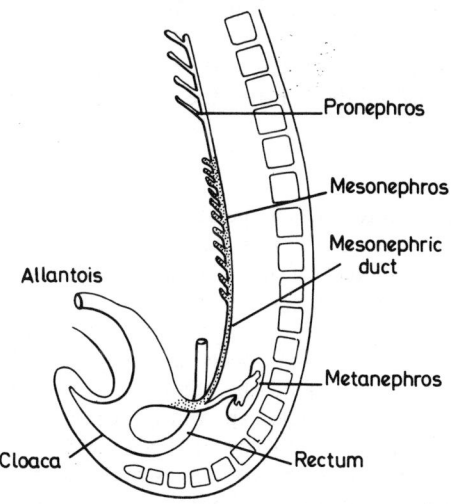

Fig. 35. A sagittal section of an embryo showing the relative positions of pronephros, mesonephros and metanephros. Note the very low position of the metanephros.

The pronephros

At about the twenty-third day of embryonic development a clump of cells appears in the mesoderm of the intermediate cell mass at the level of the ninth somite. It proliferates, and spreading downwards as a solid cord, reaches and fuses with the cloaca. Later the cord acquires a lumen, and becomes a tube which is known as the pronephric or primary excretory duct. In some species, but not in man, pronephric tubules differentiate at the upper end of the pronephric duct, and connect it to the coelomic cavity.

The mesonephros

The mesonephros appears later than and caudal to the pronephros. Cells of the mesoderm between the lower cervical and upper lumbar segments differentiate into tubules, one end of which opens into the primary excretory duct, which is now called the mesonephric duct, while the other end dilates, is invaginated by a lateral branch of the primitive aorta and becomes a glomerulus. In all, between 70 and 80 mesonephric tubules appear but as the early ones disappear before the later ones develop, no more than 30 to 40 are present at any one time. Only a few mesonephric tubules persist into adult life. They do not contribute to the urinary tract and become in the male the efferent ductules of the testis, the lobules of the head of the epididymis, and the ductules aberrantes, and in the female, the ep-oophoron and the para-oophoron.

The metanephros

The metanephros, which persists as the adult kidney, first appears when the embryo is 5 weeks old (Fig 36). A bud grows out of the lower end of the mesonephric duct into the most caudal part of the intermediate cell mass. This bud elongates to form the ureter and its blind upper end dilates to form the renal pelvis, the calyces and the collecting ducts of the kidney (Fig. 37). The mesoderm around the blind end of the ureteric bud is called the metanephrogenic cap, and gives rise to the glomeruli, the proximal tubules, the loops of Henle and the distal tubules. Eventually fusion occurs between the structures derived from the metanephrogenic cap and the collecting ducts derived from the ureteric bud.

The caudal ends of the mesonephric ducts gradually move

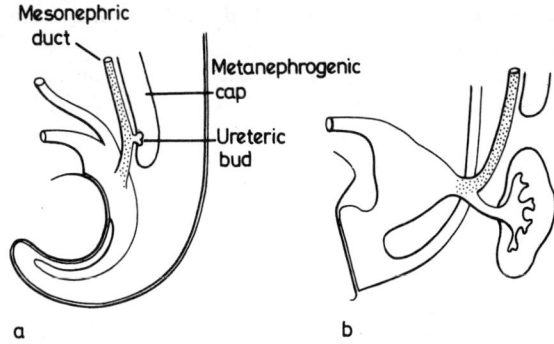

Fig. 36. Origin of the metanephros, showing the origin of the ureteric bud from the caudal end of the mesonephric duct, and of the metanephrogenic cap from the caudal part of the mesoderm of the intermediate cell mass.

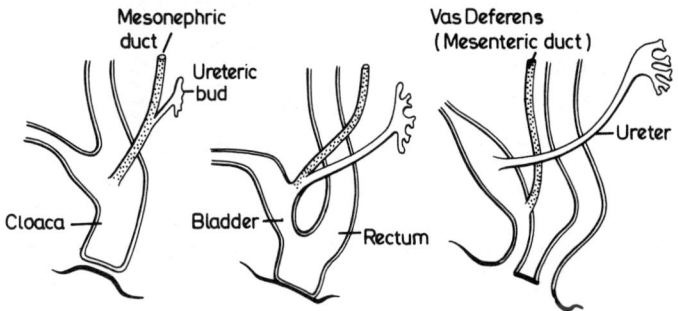

Fig. 37. Diagram showing elongation of the ureter and expansion of its upper end into renal pelvis and calyces; the manner in which the lower end of the ureter is carried downwards by the mesonephric duct and eventually opens into the bladder at the lateral angle of the trigone.

downwards, fuse in the midline and become incorporated into the cloaca to form the trigone of the bladder and the prostatic urethra. The ureters are carried downwards with the mesonephric ducts, and eventually open into the bladder at the lateral angles of the trigone. The lower ends of the mesonephric ducts open into the prostatic urethra, and become the ejaculatory ducts.

At birth, each kidney contains about one million nephrons which gradually increase in size, but not in number. The kidneys grow slowly in comparison with the rest of the body, being 1 per cent of the body weight at birth, but only 0.4 per cent of the body weight in adult life. The foetal kidney is lobulated and only

175

acquires the smooth outline of the adult kidney some 3 to 4 years after birth.

The kidney is originally a pelvic organ, but as the ureter elongates it ascends and reaches its adult position high on the posterior abdominal wall during the fifth month of intrauterine life. As it ascends, it rotates through 90°, bringing the renal pelvis, which is at first in front of the kidney, to its medial aspect (Fig. 38).

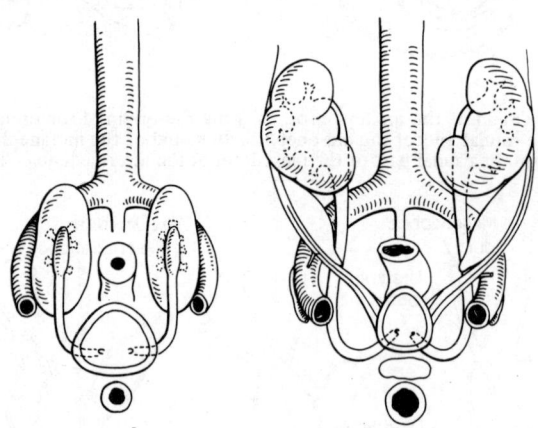

Fig. 38. The ascent and rotation of the kidneys during foetal life. Each kidney rotates through 90°, the left clockwise, the right anticlockwise.

The adult renal artery is acquired only after the kidney has ascended to the loin. Before and during its ascent, the kidney is supplied by a variety of vessels, and receives blood at one time or another from the common iliac, the internal iliac, the medial sacral and the suprarenal arteries.

Bladder

The bladder is formed in part from the caudal portion of the mesonephric duct, and in part from the cloaca. The cloaca is derived from the entoderm and is the terminal portion of the hindgut tube. It is divided by the urorectal septum into a posterior part, which forms the rectum and anus, and into an anterior part which divides into two portions, a cephalic part called the vesico-ureteric portion, and a caudal part called the urogenital sinus. The urogenital sinus forms the membranous and

176

spongy parts of the urethra in the male, and the vestibule of the vagina in the female. The vesico-ureteric portion forms the body of the bladder and the anterior wall of the prostatic urethra. The allantois, which connects the hindgut to the embryonic yolk-sac, passes from the front of the vesico-ureteric portion of the cloaca into the body stalk, and becomes the median umbilical ligament, which persists in adult life as a fibrous cord connecting the bladder to the umbilicus.

CONGENITAL ANOMALIES

About 10 per cent of people are born with one or more congenital anomalies of the urogenital tract, which vary from minor defects, which remain undetected during life, to serious abnormalities which cause death in infancy.

Anomalies of the Kidney

Congenital anomalies of the kidney can be classified as variations from normal in number, volume, structure, form, location or rotation.

Anomalies of number

Bilateral renal agenesis is very rare and is incompatible with life.

Unilateral renal agenesis occurs in 1 per 600 or 700 of the population. A kidney can be congenitally absent because the ureteric bud fails to appear and both ureter and kidney are absent, or because the metanephrogenic cap fails to differentiate and the ureter ends blindly without expanding to form pelvis or calyces, or because the mesonephric duct does not appear and not only the kidney and ureter but also the one half of the trigone and the ipsilateral genital apparatus are absent.

If one kidney is congenitally absent the other is both hypertrophied and hyperplastic and may be as long as 20 cm.

Anomalies of volume

Hypoplasia of a kidney occurs if the metanephrogenic cap differentiates, but fails to grow. Although small, a hypoplastic kidney has a distinct cortex and medulla, and functions, but not so well as a normal kidney. The ureteric bud dilates forming a pelvis and a calyceal system which are small but may otherwise be normal. Occasionally, the calyces have a clubbed appearance, and the radiological appearances may then be indistinguishable from those of chronic pyelonephritis (Fig. 39).

Hypertrophy, which is increase in size of the nephrons, occurs whenever the function of the opposite kidney is reduced by more than 20 per cent. The amount of hypertrophy depends not only on the amount function is reduced in the opposite kidney but also on the time available for its development. The normal kidney is more hypertrophied if the other is congenitally absent or hypoplastic than if it is damaged by acquired disease.

Hyperplasia, which is an increase in the number of nephrons, can only occur before birth, and therefore is only found if the other kidney is congenitally absent or hypoplastic.

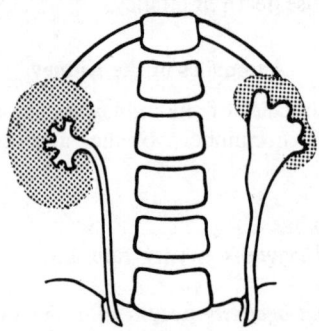

Fig. 39. A congenital hypoplastic kidney. The pelvis and calyces are dilated and the kidney is small. Most hypoplastic kidneys have a small but otherwise normal pelvi-calyceal system and lie nearer the midline than a normal kidney.

Anomalies of structure

Congenital solitary cysts. Solitary cysts may result from mal-union between a distal tubule (derived from the metanephrogenic cap) and a collecting duct (derived from the ureteric bud). Alternatively, they may arise as the result of obstruction to a renal tubule. The cysts contain clear fluid, do not communicate with the calyces and renal pelvis, and tend to be unilateral rather than bilateral. They are seldom large enough to produce abdominal swelling, but appear in pyelograms as space-occupying lesions which may be confused with tumours.

178

Congenital polycystic disease. Congenital polycystic disease occurs in 1 per 1,000 of the population; it is a Mendelian dominant trait in about 4 per cent of patients and may be associated with hepatic cystic disease or splenic cystic disease, or both. It is characterized by cystic enlargement of both kidneys, and is caused by widespread failure of fusion between collecting tubules derived from the ureteric bud, and renal tubules derived from the metanephrogenic cap. The cysts, which are always bilateral, are cortical, and are filled with clear fluid. They do not communicate with the calyces or pelvis. They compress the normal renal parenchyma, which atrophies. If the cysts are large and numerous they cause marked enlargement of both kidneys, and eventually lead to chronic renal failure. The clinical features of the disease depend on its severity. Mild cases may have no symptoms and normal renal function. Severe cases present in infancy, and moderate cases in the third, fourth or fifth decade with chronic renal failure, sometimes associated with pain, pyuria or haematuria. Both kidneys are enlarged and are usually easily palpable. The pyelographic appearances are characteristic.

Treatment is that of the chronic renal failure the disease causes, but puncture of the cysts by open operation (Rovsing's operation) sometimes relieves pain and temporarily improves renal function.

Medullary sponge kidney. This condition consists of a congenital cystic dilatation of the collecting ducts of the renal medulla. The dilatation may affect a small area of one kidney, or be widespread and bilateral. Medullary sponge disease is often symptomless, and diagnosed only on routine intravenous pyelography. The cysts, which are always tiny, may interfere with the function of the collecting ducts and with the medullary osmotic gradient, impairing renal concentrating ability and causing polyuria. The cysts frequently contain calcified deposits which may erode through into the calcyes, and pass down the ureter, causing pain and haematuria.

In early cases, intravenous pyelography may demonstrate the dilated collecting ducts. Later, medullary calcification is the most striking feature, and the calyces have a splayed appearance.

The differential diagnosis of medullary sponge kidney is from other forms of nephrocalcinosis.

Anomalies of form

Foetal lobulation. Lobulated at birth, the kidney acquires a smooth outline by the age of 4 or 5 years. Foetal lobulation persists into adult life in about 4 per cent of the population, but it is of no clinical importance.

Renal fusion. Two types of renal fusion can occur, contralateral, called a horseshoe kidney, and ipsilateral, called a sigmoid kidney.

In a horseshoe kidney, each renal segment lies on its correct side of the midline (Fig. 40), but they are joined at their lower or, less often, upper poles, by an isthmus which may be a band of renal parenchyma, or simply a strand of fibrous tissue.

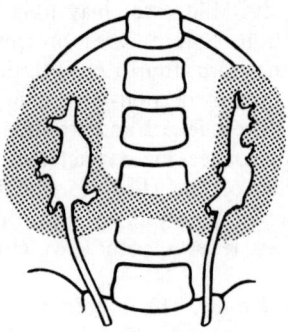

Fig. 40. A horseshoe kidney in which the lower poles of the kidneys are joined together by an isthmus of renal parenchyma. Neither kidney has rotated and the pelves are anterior.

In sigmoid or S-shaped kidney the lower pole of one kidney is joined to the upper pole of the other, and both lie on the same side of the midline. Both ureters enter the bladder normally, but one takes a devious course across the midline in order to do so (Fig. 41).

Fused kidneys rarely ascend as high as normal ones, and often fail to rotate. They are more prone than normal kidneys to infection, stone and obstruction.

Anomalies of location

Congenital renal ectopia (Fig. 42). An ectopic kidney is one that has failed to ascend to the loin and remains in the pelvis. If both kidneys are ectopic they are usually fused. An ectopic

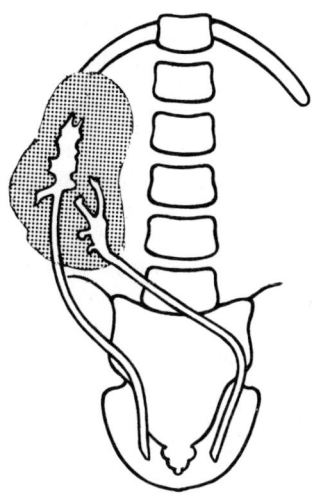

Fig. 41. A sigmoid kidney, in which the upper pole of one kidney is joined to the lower pole of the other. Both lie on the same side of the midline.

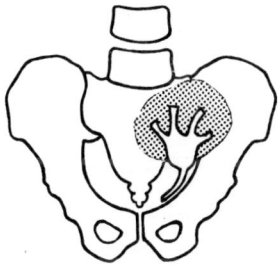

Fig. 42. An ectopic left kidney. Note the horizontal lie of the kidney and the short ureter.

kidney has a short ureter and usually fails to rotate. The normal renal artery appears only after the kidney has ascended to the loin, and an ectopic kidney therefore has an abnormal blood supply which may be derived from practically any neighbouring vessel.

Abnormal renal mobility (nephroptosis). Nephroptosis is a condition of adult life and not a true congenital abnormality. It is usually found in thin female patients, many of whom suffer from faulty nutrition and psychoneurosis. The ureter is of normal length, but the kidney has unusually long blood vessels. In the supine position the kidney lies in the loin, but it descends an abnormal distance when the patient stands and the ureter may become kinked, causing renal pain. The long arteries of the nephroptopic kidney are sometimes so stretched when the kidney descends that transient ischaemia occurs and interferes with renal function. The operation to fix a nephroptopic kidney is called nephropexy. Patients with nephroptosis tend to have numerous symptoms in addition to those which can be attributed to undue renal mobility, and in most, psychogenic complaints appear to be more prominent than those which have an organic basis. Nephropexy should be advised only if there is pain or altered renal function which can definitely be attributed to nephroptosis.

Anomalies of rotation (Fig. 43)

At first, the renal pelvis lies anterior to the kidney. As the kidney ascends to the loin the pelvis rotates through 90° and eventually takes up a medial position. Kidneys which fail to ascend (i.e. fused and ectopic kidneys) fail to rotate. Failure of rotation may also occur in kidneys which are quite normal in structure and position. If this abnormality is not kept in mind, the rather odd-looking pyelogram produced by this anomaly may be attributed to acquired disease. Treatment is not required for malrotation alone.

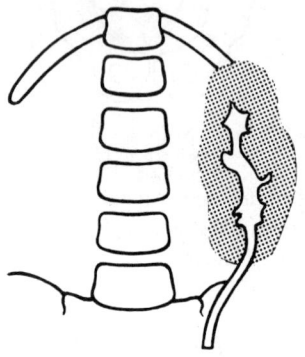

Fig. 43. A malrotated but otherwise normal kidney. The pelvis and pelvi-ureteric junction lie anteriorly and some of the calyces face med-ially. In a normally rotated kidney all the calyces face upwards, downwards or laterally.

Anomalies of the Renal Pelvis

Duplication

The blind upper end of the ureteric bud dilates to form the renal pelvis. This branches and gives rise to the superior, medial and inferior major calyces, each of which subdivides into minor calyces. The precise arrangement of the pelvis and calyces is not constant, and bizarre appearances are commonly found in pyelograms of kidneys that are otherwise normal. No less than 10 per cent of pelves appear bifid because they divide into two instead of three major calyces. A double, or duplex, kidney occurs when the ureteric bud splits after entering the metanephrogenic cap and forms two pelves. It is to be distinguished from the extremely rare anomaly in which two quite separate kidneys are found on one side. Duplicated pelves are usually situated one above the other, and are readily detected in pyelograms. They cause symptoms only if they become the site of obstruction, infection or stone formation, and are no more liable to such complications than normal kidneys.

Congenital hydronephrosis

Hydronephrosis is dilatation of the pelvis and calyces of the kidney. It can be caused by a defect in the muscle of the pelvi-ureteric junction which prevents transmission of the contraction wave and consequently interferes with the passage of urine. Since the muscular defect is an inborn error, hydronephrosis of this type is known as congenital hydronephrosis. About 60 per cent of patients with congenital hydronephrosis have an aberrant renal artery to the lower pole of the kidney, which can compress the renal pelvis and aggravate the condition. There is some difference of opinion whether or not some cases of congenital hydronephrosis are caused by aberrant vessels alone.

Congenital hydronephrosis causes incomplete obstruction to the outflow of urine from the pelvis, and although it predisposes to infection and stones, often causes few symptoms apart from mild pain, aggravated by drinking.

Treatment is surgical, and consists of pyeloplasty (Fig. 44). If the kidney is severely infected, if it contains stones, or if back pressure has caused marked thinning of the cortex, nephrectomy may be the better operation, provided that the other kidney is normal.

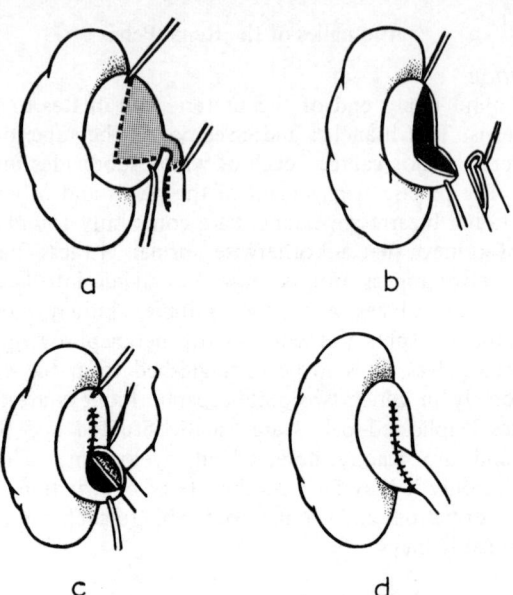

Fig. 44. Diagrams to illustrate the Anderson-Hynes pyeloplasty for congenital hydronephrosis. a. Excision of the pelvi-ureteric junction and redundant pelvis. b. Fashioning of the upper ureter. c. The pelvis has been closed and the new pelvi-ureteric junction is being sutured. d. Completed operation showing the wide dependent and spouted pelvi-ureteric junction.

Anomalies of vessels

The kidney may be supplied by aberrant arteries arising from the renal artery or the aorta. The most common abnormality is an aberrant artery passing to the lower pole of the kidney across the anterior aspect of the pelvi-ureteric junction, which aggravates and may sometimes cause congenital hydronephrosis. Ectopic kidneys derive their blood supply from vessels in their immediate vicinity.

The Ureters

Anomalies of number

Failure of one or both ureteric buds to appear is always accompanied by renal agenesis.

Ureteral duplication. Ureteral duplication is a common

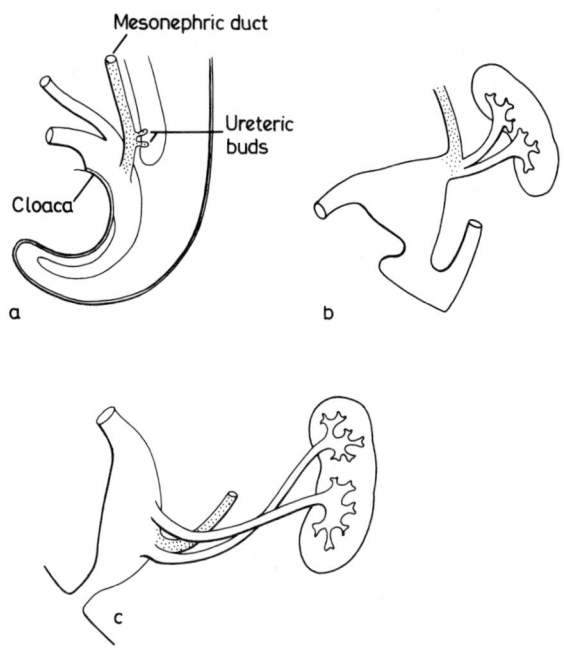

Fig. 45. Complete ureteral duplication. Two ureteric buds appear one above the other. Each elongates and forms a pelvi-calyceal system. As the mesonephric duct descends, the lower ureteric bud reaches the bladder first and opens at the lateral angle of the trigone. The upper ureteric bud is carried downwards and opens at a lower level than the lower one.

malformation and may be unilateral or bilateral, complete or incomplete. If two ureteral buds appear there will be two complete ureters, and the pelves and calyces will be duplex. The ureter from the lower pelvis always enters the bladder at a higher level than the ureter from the upper pelvis (Fig. 45). A single ureteric bud may split into two at any level. If this occurs, the pelvis is duplex but the two ureters join each other before entering the bladder. Approximately 25 per cent of patients with ureteral duplication have other abnormalities, which include renal agenesis, renal hypoplasia, polycystic disease, malrotation, ectopic ureters and renal fusion.

Ectopic ureter

An ectopic ureter is one that opens at some point other than the lateral angle of the vesical trigone. The condition is three times as common in females as in males. During development, the ureter is carried down by the mesonephric duct and if it fails to open in its normal position at the lateral angle of the trigone, it may open at any site in the tissues formed by the caudal end of the mesonephric duct. In males, the ectopic orifice always lies above the external sphincter, and incontinence does not occur, but in females the ectopic ureter usually opens into the urethra below the external sphincter or into the vagina and incontinence occurs.

In some cases of complete ureteric duplication, one ureter enters the bladder normally but the second is ectopic.

Ureterocele

A ureterocele is a cystic dilatation of the lower end of the ureter which bulges into the bladder. All layers of the ureter are involved in the cyst, which is covered by vesical mucosa separated by a few muscle fibres from the ureteric mucosa. A ureterocele is associated with an abnormally small ureteric orifice, which may be the cause of ureterocele.

Retrocaval ureter

The ureter normally lies anterior to the great vessels, and crosses in front of the common iliac vein. If the inferior vena cava develops from the lateral instead of the medial foetal cardinal veins, it passes behind the inferior vena cava or the common iliac vein, and is called retrocaval.

Megaureter (congenital dilatation of the ureter)

This condition is analogous to congenital hydronephrosis. It is due to a muscle defect in a short segment of the ureter, usually in the lower third, which prevents normal transmission of the contraction wave and obstructs the flow of urine. The ureter is not only dilated, but elongated and tortuous.

Bladder

Numerous malformations of the bladder have been described. The most important of these are diverticulum of the bladder, exstrophy of the bladder, urachal cyst and urachal fistula.

True congenital vesical diverticulum

A true congenital vesical diverticulum is rare. Even in infants most bladder diverticula are acquired following obstruction to outflow of urine from the bladder. However, congenital diverticulum may occur either near the ureteric orifice where the entodermal cloaca joins the mesonephric duct, or from urachal remnants in the vault of the bladder (Fig. 46a).

Exstrophy of the bladder

In this condition there is an absence of the lower abdominal wall and also of the anterior wall of the bladder. As a result, the posterior wall of the bladder opens on to the surface of the body. The ureteric orifices are visible and discharge urine to the exterior. The condition may be associated with epispadias and

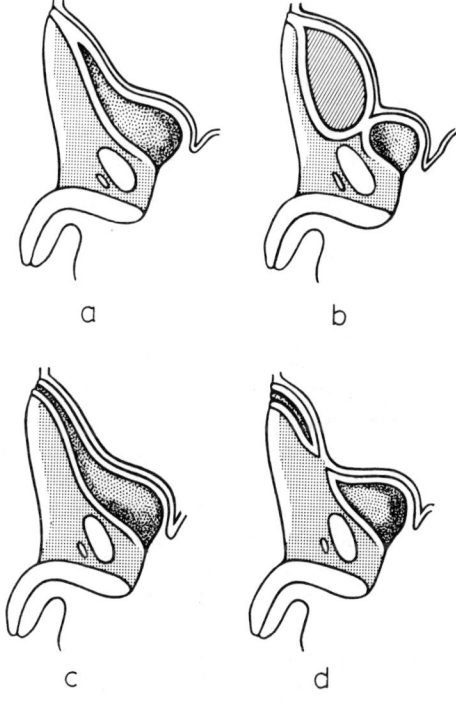

Fig. 46. Anomalies of the urachus. a. Diverticulum. b. Urachal cyst. c. Patent urachus. d. Urachal sinus.

wide separation of the pubic symphysis, or with other anomalies of the ureters or kidneys. Ascending infection occurs readily and may be fatal in the early years of life. To repair the defect in the bladder is difficult, and urine is usually diverted into the colon by a uretero-colic anastomosis.

Urachal cysts

Urachal cysts form if both ends of the urachus close but the middle remains patent. They are usually found in the lower third of the urachus, and may become so large as to be mistaken for a distended bladder (Fig. 46b).

Patent urachus

If the urachus remains patent in its whole length a urinary fistula develops between the bladder and the umbilicus (Fig. 46c).

Urethra

Congenital phimosis

Phimosis is a contracture of the prepuce sufficient to prevent its retraction over the glans. The preputial opening may be so small as to permit only a slow discharge of urine and produce severe urinary obstruction with renal damage.

Hypospadias

Hypospadias is a congenital defect of the urethra in which the external urinary meatus opens ventral and posterior to its normal position. It can be classified as glandular, penile or perineal according to the position of the meatus, which is often stenosed. The posterior urethra is never involved and incontinence does not occur because the sphincters are intact. Hypospadias occurs because the urethral groove which fuses from behind to form the urethra, closes incompletely, and it is often associated with other anomalies of the genital or urinary tract. Dilatation of the meatus usually relieves obstruction in mild cases, but extensive reconstructive surgery may be required for others.

Congenital bladder neck obstruction

Congenital hypertrophy of the verumontanum, posterior urethral valves or congenital stenosis of the bladder neck all obstruct the flow of urine from the bladder. Retention of urine occurs and is often associated with dilatation of the ureters and renal pelvis, infection and bladder diverticula. Renal failure soon follows unless the lesion is treated. Frequency is the earliest symptom and exists from birth. It is soon followed by overflow incontinence, which is often mistaken for enuresis, from the distended bladder. The distended bladder produces a large swelling which may be mistaken for an abdominal tumour, and the infant may become purple in the face while straining to pass urine. Nevertheless, symptoms are often overlooked until infection occurs. Infection of the hydronephrotic kidneys soon leads to chronic renal failure, which many of the patients already have when they first present for treatment.

Posterior urethral valves are deep folds of redundant mucosa situated in the posterior urethra and usually attached to the verumontanum. The valves are often paper thin and vary widely in position and shape. They are never imperforate although the opening may be extremely small (Fig 47).

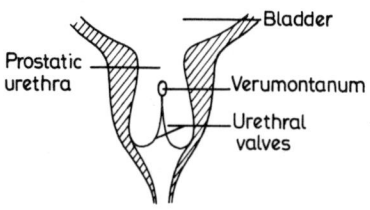

Fig. 47. Posterior urethral valves.

Congenital hypertrophy of the verumontanum (prostatic eminence). The verumontanum is two to three times its normal size. It occupies most of the urethra, sometimes extending into the bladder, and obstructs urinary outflow.

Congenital bladder neck stenosis. This is a form of congenital urethral stricture, similar to and often co-existing with congenital stenosis of the external urethral meatus. Histologically there is an increase of fibrous tissue in the submucosa. It causes less obstruction than posterior urethral valves or a hypertrophied verumontanum and therefore presents at a later age, sometimes in adults. The distended bladder and dilated ureters associated with this lesion are sometimes called megacystis and megaureter respectively.

Posterior urethral valves and hypertrophied verumontanum

occur only in males and are treated by transurethral resection. Congenital stenosis of the bladder neck can and does occur in females as well as males and may be treated either by transurethral resection or by reconstruction at open operation.

FURTHER READING

Davies, D. V. & Davies, F. (1962). *Gray's Anatomy,* 33rd ed., pp. 222 – 239. London: Longman.
Williams, D. I. (1965). In *Clinical Surgery,* Vol. 6. Ed. Fergusson, J. D. London: Butterworths.
Williams, D. I. (1968). *Paediatric Urology.* London: Butterworths.

Chapter 12

INJURIES TO THE KIDNEYS AND URINARY TRACT

INJURIES OF THE KIDNEY

The kidneys are small and mobile and are relatively well protected by muscles and viscera anteriorly, and by muscles and the lower ribs laterally and posteriorly. They are, however, liable to be damaged by gunshot or knife wounds, by severe, direct trauma from kicks or falls, or by crushing injuries, such as pedestrians sustain when run over by a vehicle. Such injuries may damage not only the kidney but also neighbouring structures like the spleen, or the liver, the ribs and the diaphragm. The damage to the kidney may consist of a subcapsular bruise, or of a laceration or lacerations involving the parenchyma. Lacerations, which may extend into the collecting system or through the capsule, may be severe enough to separate the upper or lower pole of the kidney from the rest of the viscus, or even to split the kidney into a number of fragments (Fig. 48). Sometimes the vascular pedicle rather than the kidney itself is injured and thrombosis or laceration of the renal artery or vein occurs.

The kidney is very vascular and bleeds copiously when injured, even if the injury is only a subcapsular bruise. Blood flows into the perinephric tissues causing bruising and swelling in the loin

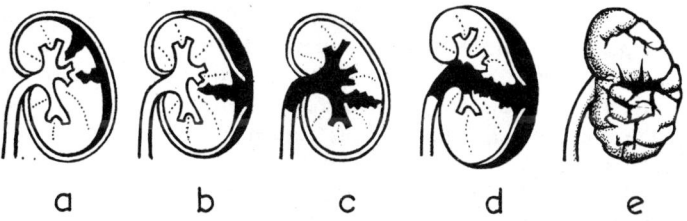

a   b   c   d   e

Fig. 48. Injury to the kidney. a. Laceration of parenchyma with sub-capsular bruise. b. Laceration of parenchyma and capsule. c. Laceration of parenchyma and calyx. d. Laceration of parenchyma, calyx and capsule. e. Fragmented kidney.

191

and into the collecting system causing haematuria. If the laceration involves the collecting system, urine may extravasate into the perinephric tissues or into the potential space between the kidney and its capsule.

Clinical features. The patient, who will have had an accident of the kind described, is usually shocked from the loss of blood and may complain of pain in the back and loin. The loin is bruised, swollen and tender and the urine contains blood, usually in amounts readily visible to the naked eye. If the damage to the kidney is only a subcapsular bruise, its function is only slightly impaired and the haematuria subsides within a few days; if the damage is more severe, its function may be markedly impaired and haematuria can persist for many days. Unless the injured kidney is a solitary one or the loss of blood causes pre-renal failure, impaired function cannot be detected by measuring the blood urea.

Treatment. Although the signs of renal injury are obvious it may be some time after the accident before they develop, and any patient who is suspected of having sustained renal damage must be admitted to hospital for observation.

Shock should be treated immediately by blood transfusion. The patient should then be examined carefully to exclude damage to neighbouring structures such as the liver, the spleen, the ribs and the diaphragm. Such injuries may not be obvious, yet if present they may be a greater danger to the patient than the renal damage.

As soon as practicable an intravenous pyelogram should be carried out. This shows whether or not the injured kidney continues to function, and whether or not the opposite kidney is normal. Sometimes an injured kidney looks surprisingly normal in the intravenous pyelogram but extravasation of dye into the perinephric tissues may be seen and, if there is bleeding into the collecting system, filling defects caused by blood clots in the pelvis and calyces.

Given time, most renal injuries heal spontaneously and can therefore be managed conservatively, but if bleeding or the extravasation of urine into the perinephric space is severe and persistent, operation has to be considered. Persistent extravasation of urine is rare, because if a kidney is so severely damaged that it

192

cannot heal itself it is usually too severely damaged to continue functioning.

URETERIC INJURIES

Severe crushing injuries or gunshot wounds may damage one or both ureters. Such injuries, however, cause widespread damage and the effects of ureteric damage tend to be overshadowed by those of damage to other viscera.

Most ureteric injuries occur during surgical operations on structures such as the uterus, the uterine cervix, the colon or the rectum. All these structures lie close to the ureters, and a ureter may be caught in a stitch or clamped and ligated along with a blood vessel. That a ureter has been injured may not be obvious immediately, unless it is solitary, or the injury is bilateral, and the patient tends to remain well for 7 or 10 days. At about this time, catgut sutures dissolve. Urine then leaks from the open end of the ureter and discharges through the wound on to the skin of the abdomen or perineum, or through the vagina, depending on the site of operation, forming a ureteric fistula. It is occasionally difficult to distinguish between a urinary and a serous discharge, especially if it is blood-stained. Any doubt about the nature of the fluid can be resolved by measuring its urea content because, even in renal failure, the concentration of urea in the urine is always at least twice its concentration in the blood. When a urinary fistula develops after operation it can be determined whether it is from the bladder or the ureter by intravenous pyelography and cystoscopy. With bladder fistulae the upper urinary tract usually remains normal and on cystoscopy the opening of the fistula into the bladder may be seen, although it is occasionally obscured by oedema. With ureteric fistulae the ureter and renal pelvis are usually dilated and dye may extravasate through the fistula. The bladder is normal. Any attempt to catheterize the ureter is usually unsuccessful because the catheter sticks at the fistula, which is usually some 5 to 10 cm above the vesico-ureteric junction.

If a solitary ureter or both ureters are ligated, the patient will have symptoms and signs of acute renal failure long before the catgut absorbs and a fistula forms. Ureteric damage must always be suspected in any patient who develops anuria immediately after a pelvic or lower abdominal operation.

Treatment

In all operations on structures close to the ureters special care should be taken to avoid damaging them. If it is realized during the operation that a ureter has been damaged, it may be possible to carry out an immediate repair by anastomosis or by reimplanting the cut proximal end of the ureter into the bladder.

If it is not realized that the ureter has been damaged until a fistula develops, a second operation must be carried out. In elderly patients whose other kidney is normal, nephrectomy may be the most satisfactory way of dealing with ureteric damage. In younger patients, and in all patients in whom there is any doubt at all about the contralateral kidney, an attempt is made to repair the damaged ureter. The site of injury is usually 5 to 10 cm above the uretero-vesical junction. It is often possible to bring the cut proximal end of the ureter downwards and reimplant it into the bladder. If this is not possible, the two cut ends are anastomosed, but this procedure is more difficult than it sounds, and frequently results in a ureteric stricture. If a solitary ureter or both ureters are involved and the patient develops anuria the obstruction must be relieved immediately by inserting a drainage tube into the kidney (nephrostomy) or into the ureter above the obstruction (ureterostomy).

INJURIES TO THE BLADDER

Injury to the bladder may cause laceration (or rupture). As the bladder fills, more and more of its surface becomes covered with peritoneum and if rupture occurs when the bladder is full, urine leaks into the peritoneal cavity, but if rupture occurs when the bladder is empty, urine leaks into the extraperitoneal tissues.

Intraperitoneal extravasation (Fig. 49a). The distended bladder may be ruptured by a hard blow on the lower abdomen, when urine leaks into the peritoneal cavity and produces the signs and symptoms of peritoneal irritation. Operation must be carried out. As much urine as possible is drained from the peritoneal cavity. The tear in the bladder is sutured, and the bladder cavity is drained for 7 or 8 days with a urethral or a supra-pubic catheter, until healing occurs.

Extraperitoneal extravasation (Fig. 49b). An empty bladder is much less liable to injury than a distended one, but it may be lacerated as the result of fractures of the pelvis, endoscopic instrumentation, or operations on pelvic viscera or femoral herniae. The urine leaks extraperitoneally, within the pelvis. On examination there is lower abdominal tenderness, usually associated with ileus. Urine is not passed per urethram, and as the bladder is empty, none is obtained on catheterization. If X-rays are taken after a radio-opaque dye is injected up the catheter, the dye is seen spreading outside the bladder. Treatment is by operation. The bladder is sutured and drained by a urethral catheter for 7 or 8 days. If the pelvis is fractured, treatment will be required for this also.

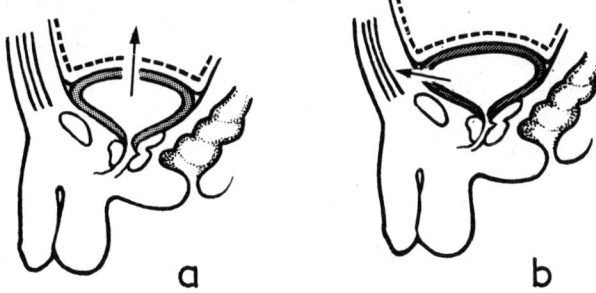

Fig. 49. Rupture of the bladder. a. Intraperitoneal. b. Extraperitoneal.

Occasionally, a malignant or tuberculous lesion of the bladder will lead to spontaneous rupture. In this case, simple suturing and drainage is insufficient, and more extensive procedures like urinary diversion or cystectomy may be required.

Bladder fistulae

A bladder fistula is a track which allows urine to leave the bladder by some route other than the urethra.

1. A vesico-cutaneous fistula connects the bladder with the skin.

2. A vesico-enteric or a vesico-colic fistula connects the bladder with the alimentary tract.

3. A vesico-uterine or vesico-vaginal fistula connects the bladder with the female genital tract.

195

Vesico-cutaneous fistula. A vesico-cutaneous fistula can arise congenitally in two ways: (a) in exstrophy of the bladder, the anterior abdominal wall is formed by the posterior wall of the bladder, and the ureters drain directly on to the body surface; (b) if the urachus persists and does not become obliterated, it forms an open tract connecting the bladder with the umbilicus (p. 188).

An acquired vesico-cutaneous fistula is usually termed a suprapubic fistula. It may arise as a complication of operations on the bladder or prostate, or be made deliberately for the relief of obstruction at the bladder neck or in the urethra.

Vesico-alimentary fistula. (a) Vesico-enteric fistula: communication between the bladder and the small bowel may develop in inflammatory disorders such as Crohn's disease, and occasionally in malignant disease. (b) Vesico-colic fistula: communication between the bladder and the large bowel, the parts of the latter involved being as a rule either rectum or sigmoid colon. It is caused more often by diverticulitis than by carcinoma, and there is usually an intervening pelvic abscess.

Faeces and flatus pass from bowel to bladder; it is unusual for urine to pass in the reverse direction. The characteristic symptom of a vesico-colic fistula is pneumaturia – the passing of flatus through the urethra at the end of micturition. Organisms also pass from the large bowel into the bladder and produce cystitis, which may be severe. It is rather strange how often diverticulitis which is severe enough to produce a fistula causes few, if any, colonic symptoms.

Vesico-genital fistula. Communication may occur between the bladder and the vagina or between the bladder and the uterus; these conditions are known as vesico-vaginal fistula and vesico-uterine fistula respectively. Damage to the bladder and genital tract leading to fistula formation can occur as the result of difficult gynaecological or obstetric procedures, by prolonged or difficult labour, or as a complication of carcinoma of the cervix or uterus. Vesico-genital fistulae lead to continuous or intermittent leakage of urine from the genital tract.

URETHRAL INJURY

Injury to the female urethra

Difficult and protracted labour is the commonest cause of

injuries to the female urethra and with adequate antenatal care and careful management of labour, such injuries can usually be prevented. Urethral injuries in the female heal without difficulty, but fibrosis may deform and distort the normal structure of the urethra, and cause stress incontinence.

Injury to the male urethra

Injuries to the male urethra may involve the membranous part (intrapelvic) or spongy part (extrapelvic), and are usually caused by accidental trauma. The urethra may, however, be damaged during instrumentation especially when metal catheters, cystoscopes, resectoscopes or lithotrites are used. A soft rubber or portex catheter rarely if ever harms the urethra, unless it is very large. Occasionally the urethra is damaged when foreign bodies or chemical solutions are introduced into it by patients who attempt to cure themselves of urethritis or urinary retention.

Membranous urethra (intrapelvic). Damage to the membranous urethra only occurs with severe trauma to the pelvis and therefore is usually associated with pelvic fracture, damage to pelvic viscera, and rupture of some of the vessels of the prostatic venous plexus. The urethra is usually completely divided, and the bladder and prostate are displaced backwards. Any urine passed extravasates into the extrapelvic tissues but fortunately the urethra tends to remain closed and urine may not be passed until it overflows from a distended bladder. The patient is often shocked and may require blood transfusion before operation. Treatment is difficult because the two ends of the urethra are widely separated and there is much bleeding. To find the two cut ends of the urethra is by no means easy, and to anastomose them usually impossible. A blunt probe known as a sound is passed through the distal urethral segment from the external meatus, and a second sound is passed outwards from the internal meatus after the bladder has been exposed and opened. A Foley catheter is then negotiated from the external meatus into the bladder, and its balloon is inflated within the bladder. Traction applied to the catheter draws the cut ends of the urethra into apposition. The traction is maintained for 10 to 14 days, and during this period the bladder is drained supra-pubically and kept empty. By the end of this period the urethra should have healed in continuity. Because of the nature of the injury and the difficulty involved in its treatment fibrosis and stricture formation almost invariably occur and the urethra has to be regularly dilated for an indefinite period.

Spongy urethra (extrapelvic). Although injury to the spongy urethra may be caused by fractures of the bony pelvis or by endoscopic instrumentation, it is more often damaged by the direct trauma of kicks or falls astride a fence or plank. The injury may consist of bruising or of partial or complete transection (rupture). A damaged urethra bleeds. Some blood escapes into the perineum and causes bruising and swelling, and some enters the urethra and leaks from the external meatus in a continuous flow. The more severe the damage to the urethra, the more it bleeds and therefore the amount of urethral bleeding and the extent of perineal bruising enable us to form some opinion about the nature of the injury. A partial rupture is more severe than bruising, but less severe than a complete rupture. The external sphincter goes into spasm, and retention of urine occurs. If urine does enter the urethra, and it is unlikely to do so until it overflows from the distended bladder, it extravasates into the superficial perineal space, which is bounded by the attachments of the membranous layer of superficial fascia, to the back of the perineal membrane and to the deep fascia of the thigh just below the inguinal ligament. Patients with injuries of the spongy urethra rarely lose sufficient blood to be shocked.

Under strict aseptic precautions in an operating theatre, an attempt is made to pass a soft urethral catheter into the bladder. If the catheter passes easily into the bladder it may be left in for 7 to 10 days, in order to prevent the extravasation of urine, and to limit the amount of fibrosis and narrowing at the site of the injury. Some surgeons prefer not to leave a catheter in the urethra and instead drain the bladder with a supra-pubic catheter. They believe that leaving a catheter in an injured urethra increases the risk of stricture formation.

If a catheter cannot be passed into the bladder, it is presumed that the urethra has been completely divided, and operation is necessary. A perineal incision is made. If it is not possible to identify the two cut ends of the urethra, one sound is passed through the external meatus and a second through the internal meatus, after exposing and opening the bladder. When repairing the urethra, only the dorsal halves of the cut ends are sutured together. A catheter is then passed through the urethra into the bladder, but the bladder is kept empty by a second catheter inserted supra-pubically. As much extravasated urine as possible is removed through two or more incisions into the superficial perineal pouch.

Rupture of the spongy urethra is less likely to be followed by fibrosis and stricture formation than rupture of the membranous urethra. Nevertheless, urethral dilatation should be carried out 1 month and 3 months after operation, and as often thereafter as seems necessary.

FURTHER READING

Baines, G. H. (1965). In *Clinical Surgery,* Vol. 6. Ed. Fergusson, J. D. London: Butterworths.
McNair, T. J. (1967). *Emergency Surgery,* 8th ed., pp. 750–762, and 783–791. Bristol: Wright.

Chapter 13

THE PROSTATE, SEMINAL VESICLES AND URETHRA

THE PROSTATE

Anatomy

The prostate gland, a primary male sex gland, is perforated by the prostatic urethra from its base, which is continuous with the bladder neck, to its apex, which rests on the deep fascia covering the deep perineal pouch. It has an inner zone which consists of glands in the mucosa and the submucosa of the prostatic urethra, and an outer zone which consists of the main prostatic glands (Fig. 50). The outer zone is adherent to the true fibrous capsule which separates it from loose pelvic fascia and the prostatic venous plexus. For descriptive purposes, the prostate may be divided into five lobes: one anterior, which is fibrous and has few, if any, glands; two lateral, which are mainly inner zone glands but have a thin rim of outer zone glands; one middle, which is all inner zone glands; and one posterior, which is nearly all outer zone glands (Fig. 51).

Because the prostate is so closely related to the bladder neck and to the urethra, prostatic infection, neoplasia, hyperplasia and fibrosis all tend to disturb micturition.

Infections

Acute prostatic infections

Acute prostatitis is usually seen in men between the ages of 30 and 50, but may complicate benign prostatic hypertrophy and therefore occur in older men. The micro-organisms are usually coliforms, especially *E. coli*, sometimes proteus or staphylococci, and rarely gonococci or streptococci. They may travel to the prostate from a distant focus by the blood stream or spread directly into it from the posterior urethra and the inflammation they cause may resolve, proceed to abscess formation or become chronic. Infection may spread to the seminal vesicles, to the

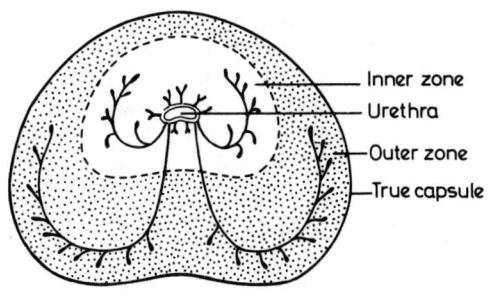

Fig. 50. Transverse section of the prostate gland.

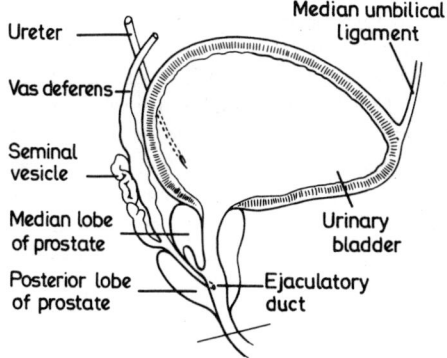

Fig. 51. Sagittal section of the bladder and prostate.

epididymis, to the bladder and kidneys and occasionally into the blood stream.

Clinical features. Acute infection of the prostate gland causes symptoms similar to those of cystitis, with which it is often confused. The onset is sudden. Malaise, vague muscle pains, fever and sometimes rigors, precede or coincide with frequent, painful and urgent micturition. There is discomfort and pain over the sacrum, in the perineum, in the supra-pubic region and in the rectum. There may be terminal haematuria, strangury, difficult micturition and even urinary retention. If an abscess forms, pain becomes throbbing and fever and other symptoms persist or increase in severity. The infected prostate is large, tender and firm, but becomes soft and fluctuant if an abscess forms. The urine remains sterile unless the posterior urethra is also infected, or an abscess ruptures into the urethra.

Treatment. Antibiotics are given because they speed resolution and may prevent the infection from spreading. To culture the organisms, and test their sensitivities to antibiotics, may be difficult because the urine is often sterile. Nevertheless a midstream specimen of urine should be obtained. Prostatic massage, which may release enough secretion into the urethra for bacteriological examination, may exacerbate the infection and even cause septicaemia. Ampicillin or oxytetracycline are given together with oestrogens, which reduce prostatic congestion and relieve symptoms. If an abscess forms it should be drained by the perineal or retro-pubic route.

Chronic prostatic infections

Chronic infections of the prostate are caused by the same types of organisms that are responsible for acute infections. They may begin as acute infections which fail to resolve, or be insidious from the outset, and may spread to involve the bladder, the kidneys or the epididymes. Symptoms vary but usually include frequent, urgent, painful, difficult micturition and sometimes urinary retention. There may also be systemic disturbance with recurrent fevers and vague ill-health. The chronically infected prostate may be only slightly enlarged, but is irregular and firm and if it contains stones, it may be so hard as to suggest malignancy. Treatment is not easy. The organism concerned can rarely be cultured from the urine, but midstream specimens of urine should nevertheless be examined. Antibiotics are usually given but are not always effective. If the urethra is obstructed, parts of the infected gland may be removed. The local symptoms and signs of tuberculous prostatitis are similar to those of non-specific chronic prostatitis, but it is always associated with tuberculous infection elsewhere in the urinary or the genital tracts, or in both (p. 136).

Simple (Benign or Senile) Enlargement of the Prostate

Although simple enlargement of the prostate is most often found in men over 60 years of age, it sometimes occurs in the sixth and even fifth decades. It is usually attributed to the endocrine changes of ageing, but no one has clearly demonstrated that the reduced androgen production and increased oestrogen production which occur in elderly males is exaggerated or otherwise altered in patients with prostatic hypertrophy, and the aetiology of the disease remains obscure.

The pathological changes of prostatic hypertrophy are confined to the inner zone glands of the lateral lobes, of the middle lobe or of both, and consist of an increase in the number of glands (adenosis) and in their cellularity (epitheliosis), an increase also in the amount of fibrous tissue in the stroma between the glands and the formation of small cysts if the ducts of the glands are blocked. (The histological changes closely resemble those of fibro-adenosis in the female breast.) If adenosis and cyst formation predominate, the inner zone enlarges, sometimes to a remarkable extent, forming one or more 'adenomata'. The hypertrophied inner zone compresses the outer zone of glands which forms a false capsule, and compresses, distorts and elongates the prostatic urethra so that the outflow of urine from the bladder is obstructed (Fig. 52). If fibrosis predominates, the gland is firmer but no larger than normal. Nevertheless a fibrosed gland may cause as much obstruction to the outflow of urine from the bladder as a large gland, because it contracts and compresses the urethra.

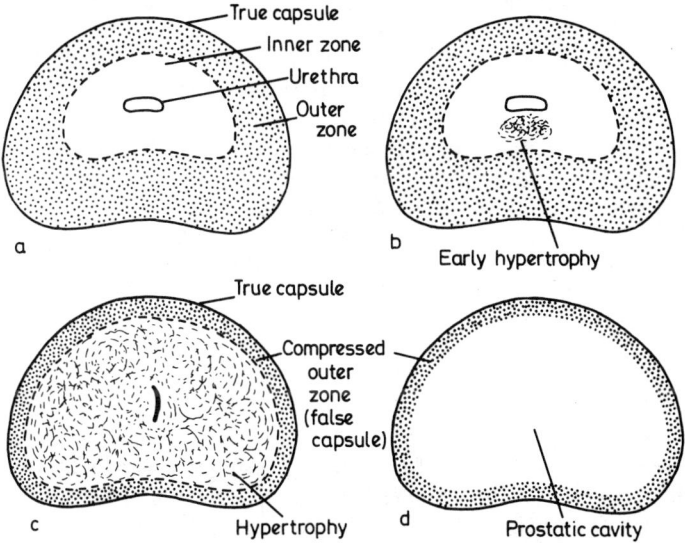

Fig. 52. Benign hypertrophy of the prostate. a. Normal gland. b. Early hypertrophy. c. Marked hypertrophy. d. After prostatectomy.

With prostatic hypertrophy as with all other lesions that obstruct the flow of urine from the bladder, secondary pathological changes may occur in the bladder, ureters and kidneys. In the bladder these changes consist of trabeculation, and sometimes of infection, stone and diverticula formation; in the upper urinary tract they consist of dilatation of the ureters and pelves (caused by back pressure but sometimes aggravated by vesico-ureteric reflux), infection, stones and chronic renal failure.

Clinical features

The clinical features of benign prostatic enlargement are those of obstruction to the outflow of urine from the bladder:

Progressive difficulty with micturition

Patients complain of difficulty in starting micturition and of increased frequency (especially at night). There is a thin, weak, urinary stream with terminal dribbling, and micturition takes a long time. The patient feels that he has not emptied the bladder.

Acute retention of urine

The patient has an urgent desire to micturate, but is unable to do so and the bladder is distended, tender and tense.

Infection, infarction or congestion may suddenly increase the size of a hypertrophied gland and cause acute urinary retention in patients who have had little, if any, previous trouble with micturition. Infarction is found in some 25 per cent of hypertrophied glands, and strangely enough it induces squamous metaplasia of the adjacent epithelium. Congestion may be caused by infection, by long journeys during which the patient has suppressed micturition, by congestive cardiac failure, in which venous congestion causes swelling not only of the liver, the spleen and the lungs, but also of the prostate, by operations on structures near the prostate, or by endoscopic procedures involving the urethra.

Chronic retention

Each time the patient micturates evacuation is incomplete and the bladder gradually but progressively distends. The patient may be unaware that his bladder is distended, but usually complains that he has little control over the small quantities of urine which overflow down the urethra at frequent intervals. Chronic retention indicates severe and prolonged obstruction and is often associated with dilatation of the upper urinary tract, vesico-ureteric reflux, infection and chronic renal failure.

Recurrent or persistent infections and stones

The patient may present with symptoms and signs of recurrent or persistent infections or of stones in the bladder and sometimes in the kidneys.

Chronic renal failure

Some patients pay little attention to difficulties with micturition or even to chronic retention, and seek advice only when they have chronic renal failure.

Haematuria

Haematuria or urethral bleeding may occur when the prostate gland is congested, and sometimes is the only symptom of prostatic hypertrophy.

Obstruction to the outflow of urine from the bladder is diagnosed from (a) the patient's history, (b) examination of the abdomen, (c) renal function tests (including intravenous pyelograms), and (d) the estimation of the amount of residual urine. In prostatic hypertrophy, the findings on rectal examination vary, depending on which lobe or lobes of the prostate are involved. If the lateral lobes are involved, the prostate feels large and smooth, is elastic and uniform in consistence, and mobile. If the middle lobe alone is affected, the prostate feels normal on rectal examination because an enlarged middle lobe projects forwards into the bladder, not backwards into the rectum, and can be recognized only by cystoscopy (Fig. 53). If the prostate is fibrous it is normal or only slightly enlarged in size but firm in consistence.

Treatment

Benign prostatic hypertrophy is treated not because the gland is large but because it is causing obstruction. Many small glands cause obstruction and many large ones do not and there is little correlation between the size of the prostate assessed by rectal examination and the degree of obstruction.

The symptoms of obstruction may be aggravated or precipitated by drugs such as propantheline, hyoscine-N-butylbromide, imipramine hydrochloride or amitryptyline hydrochloride, which all relax smooth muscle and may reduce the strength of bladder contraction.

Medical treatment (e.g. oestrogens or antibiotics) may reduce congestion in the gland, control infection and improve renal function and the patient's general condition. Such measures, however, will have little effect on the changes of benign prostatic hypertrophy, which can be treated only by the operation of prostatectomy.

Fifty per cent of patients in the age group that have prostatic hypertrophy suffer from one or more of such diseases as chronic bronchitis, angina, hypertension, diabetes or previous coronary thrombosis. At one time, such patients had to put up with what

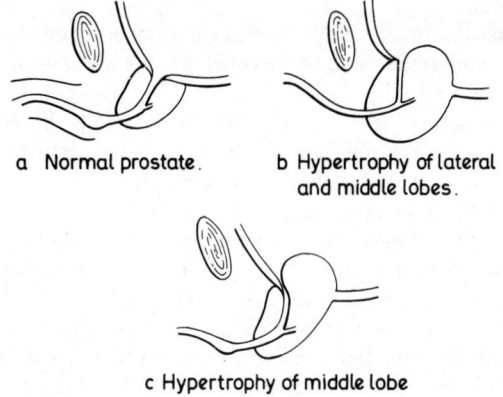

a Normal prostate.   b Hypertrophy of lateral and middle lobes.

c Hypertrophy of middle lobe

Fig. 53. Prostatic hypertrophy.

urinary difficulties they suffered or be treated by the insertion of a supra-pubic catheter, which relieved the patient of urinary obstruction, but condemned him to permanent infection and an uneasy symbiosis with a smelly urinal. With modern anaesthetic techniques, few (if any) patients must be condemned to this kind of existence because the risks of prostatectomy even in the frailest and oldest patients are slight.

The management of benign prostatic hypertrophy depends upon the signs and symptoms with which the patient presents and upon the patient's general health (Figs. 54, 55 and 56).

In those patients who have retention, recurrent infections, stones or chronic renal failure, the need for treatment is obvious.

In others to decide whether or not treatment is required can be difficult. If the patient complains only of increased frequency it must be made quite sure that his symptoms are caused by obstruction and not by uninhibited or voluntary neurogenic bladder (p. 247), or by polyuria. This can be done by looking for the effects of obstruction in the bladder (trabeculation, diverticulum, residual urine) or in upper urinary tract. Frequency unless accompanied by difficulty in starting and stopping micturition and by a diminution in the force and calibre of the urinary stream is probably not caused by obstruction. It is not how often the patient passes urine that is important but how long it takes him to do so.

Drainage of the bladder always improves renal function if it is reduced by chronic retention, and may restore it to normal if

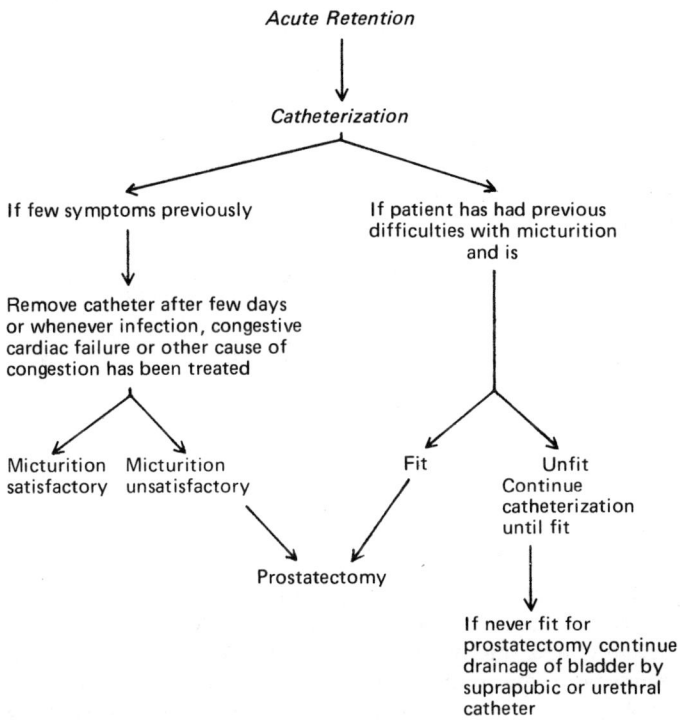

Fig. 54. Management of acute retention.

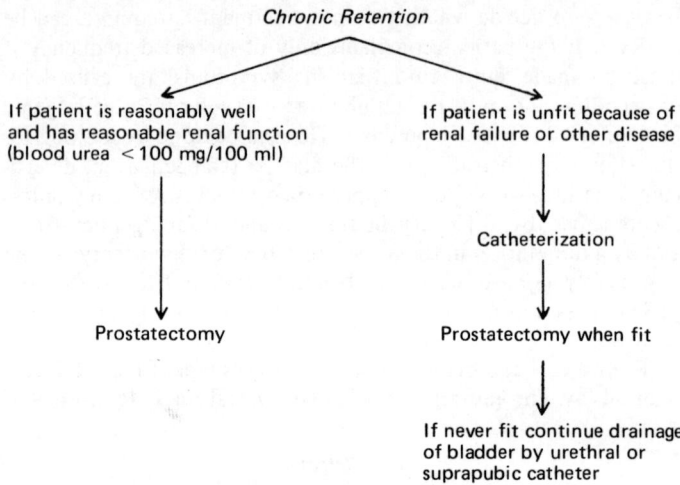

Fig. 55. Management of chronic retention.

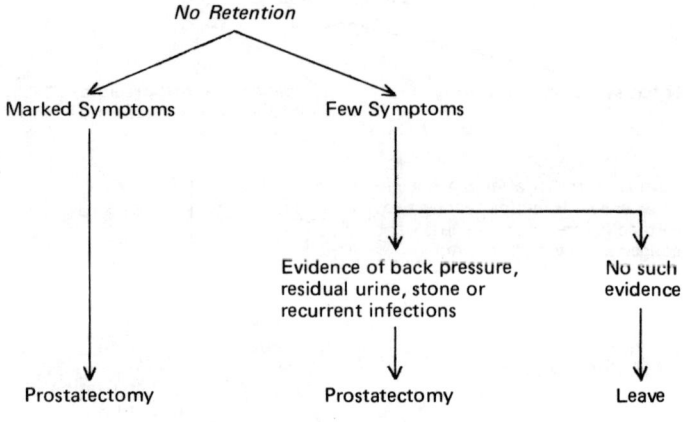

Fig. 56. Management without retention.

there is little, or no, parenchymatous destruction. Peritoneal dialysis and haemodialysis do nothing to relieve obstruction, and therefore have no place in the management of chronic renal failure caused by prostatic hypertrophy except perhaps to keep a moribund patient alive until conservative measures such as catheterization have had time to work.

It is sometimes argued that patients with prostatic hypertrophy should be operated on early, even if symptoms are few, because this will avoid operation some years later when the patient is older and less fit. This is a specious argument, however, because symptoms of prostatic hypertrophy are not always progressive, and a patient may be no more in need of an operation 10 years hence than he is now.

A congested hypertrophied prostate may cause haematuria or urethral bleeding, but haematuria must never be attributed to prostatic congestion, no matter how large the prostate, until some more serious lesion in the upper or lower urinary tract has been excluded. Unless severe, haematuria alone is not an indication for prostatectomy.

At operation for benign prostatic hypertrophy only the hypertrophied part of the gland is removed. The compressed outer group of glands (sometimes called the false capsule) and the true prostatic capsule are left intact (Fig. 52). The hypertrophied part can easily be enucleated from the false capsule, unless it is fibrous. The prostate gland can be approached by five different routes: transvesical, retro-pubic, transurethral, perineal or sacral, but only the first three of these are used in this country. By whichever route the prostate is approached, the principles of the operation are (1) to enucleate or resect the hypertrophied part of the gland from the false capsule without damaging adjacent structures, (2) to obtain reasonable haemostasis in the prostatic cavity, (3) to drain blood from the bladder before it clots, and (4) to avoid infection. The raw prostatic cavity becomes lined by epithelium in 7 to 10 days. Large glands are best dealt with by transvesical or retro-pubic operation, small fibrous ones by transurethral resection (Fig. 57).

Some believe that transurethral resection must be simpler and safer than open prostatectomy and therefore ideal for those patients who seem unfit for open operation. However, transurethral resection involves as much manipulation, time, anaesthesia and blood loss as an open operation, and if the patient is fit for the one he is fit for the other. Whether transurethral or open prostatectomy is carried out depends on the condition of the prostate, not on the condition of the patient.

Carcinoma of the Prostate

Carcinoma of the prostate, which is an adenocarcinoma, starts in the outer zone glands of a normal or hypertrophied prostate, and may occur in the false capsule deliberately left behind after prostatectomy for benign hypertrophy. It grows directly through the true prostatic capsule into the peri-prostatic tissues, and spreads into the trigone of the bladder, obstructing the ureters, and around but rarely into the rectum. It also spreads along lymphatic channels to the lymph nodes along the internal iliac vessels, and by the blood vessels, particularly the vertebral system of veins, to the lumbar vertebrae, the bony pelvis and the upper femora.

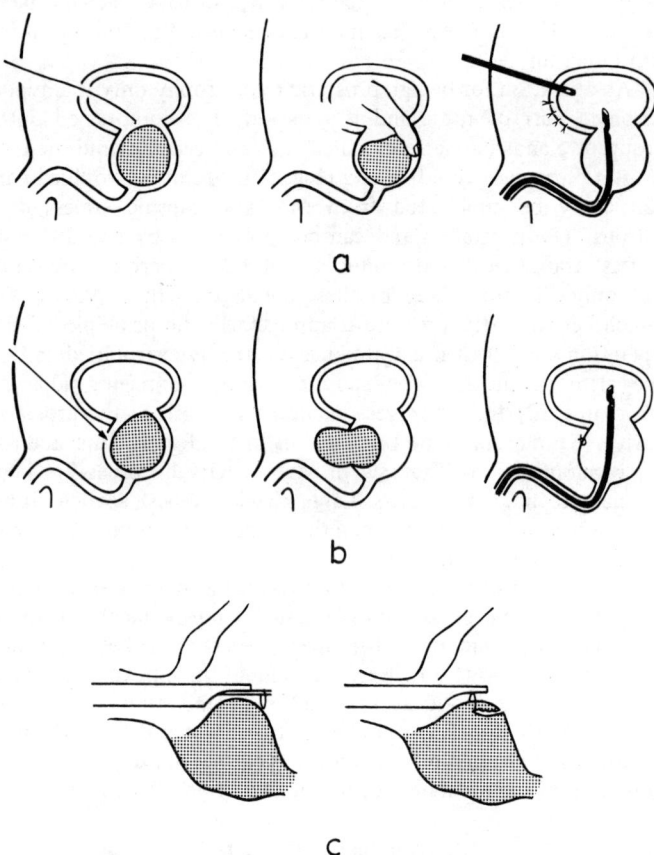

Fig. 57. Prostatectomy. a. Transvesical. b. Retropubic. c.Transurethral.

Bony metastases, unlike those of other tumours, are osteo-blastic and appear in X-rays as sclerotic areas.

Clinical features

If the malignant gland obstructs the urethra, the patient complains of difficulties in micturition, urinary retention, infection, stones or chronic renal failure, indistinguishable from those caused by benign enlargement. Because carcinoma begins in outer zone glands it only obstructs the urethra when it is locally advanced, and some patients have few, if any, urinary symptoms but complain instead of pain in the back or sciatica caused by bony metastases. On rectal examination the malignant gland feels hard, irregular and fixed, and its median furrow is usually obliterated. The disease may extend out to the side walls of the pelvis, around the rectum, and under, and sometimes into the trigone of the bladder. The serum acid phosphatase may be raised, especially when the disease has spread through the capsule or into the bones, or both, but a normal acid phosphatase is consistent with the diagnosis of carcinoma. Biopsy, which is usually carried out transrectally, carries risks but is sometimes done if the diagnosis is in doubt.

Carcinoma of the prostate rarely, if ever, causes symptoms until it has spread beyond the capsule and is incurable by radical surgery. Few, if any, patients are therefore suitable for radical surgery. The tumour is relatively radio-resistant, and treatment is based on hormonal therapy. The normal prostate depends on androgens for its proper growth and function, and so do some carcinomas of the prostate. Androgenic secretion can be signi-ficantly reduced by orchidectomy or by giving large doses of oestrogens, or by both. One method of treatment is to carry out an orchidectomy (usually as a testicular evisceration in which the seminiferous tubules of both testes are scooped out from the tunica albuginea, which is left behind), and to give dienoestrol 45 mg or ethinyloestradiol 3 mg daily. If the patient is old or frail, operation may be omitted and only oestrogens given. Such large amounts of oestrogens invariably cause gynaecomastia, and some-times cause nausea and vomiting which may be so severe that it becomes necessary to reduce the dose of oestrogens or even stop them altogether. Oestrogens may cause fluid retention and even oedema, and must be used with caution in patients who have heart disease or hypertension.

Honvan is phosphorylated stilboestrol and has no oestrogenic effects. If given orally or by injection it is dephosphorylated in the prostate and in prostatic metastases, and releases stilboestrol, which is an active oestrogen, in the places it is most needed. Unfortunately, much of the ingested or injected Honvan is altered in the liver or bound by serum protein and it is little, if any, better than ordinary oestrogens.

The adrenal glands produce androgens under the influence of ACTH from the anterior pituitary. Adrenalectomy or hypophysectomy has been carried out in patients with carcinomas of the prostate that have failed to respond to or escaped from oestrogens but the results are disappointing (Fig. 58). If the patient has serious difficulties with micturition and they do not improve with hormonal therapy, part of the prostate can be removed by transurethral resection.

Prostatic Calculi

True prostatic calculi (not to be confused with false 'prostatic' calculi which come from the bladder and lodge in the posterior urethra), develop in stagnant or infected acini as the result of deposition of calcareous material on the corpora amylacea (small bodies of amorphous debris and desquamated epithelium which lie in the acini of the prostatic glands), and are usually found in men

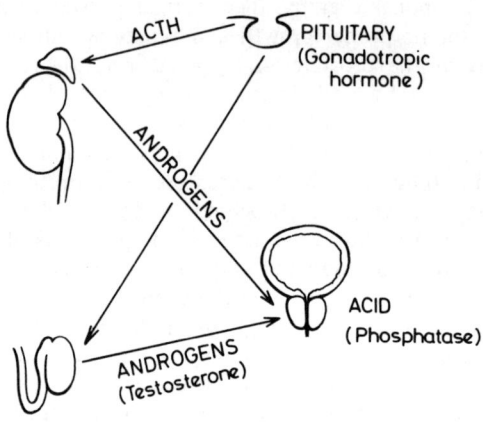

Fig. 58. Hormones acting upon the prostate.

between the ages of 50 and 65. They are generally small and multiple, and found in infected glands or in the compressed outer zone of a gland involved in benign hypertrophy.

Calculi themselves rarely cause symptoms, and are found only on X-ray examination or during prostatectomy for senile hypertrophy. The clinical features of prostatic calculi are those of the associated simple hypertrophy or chronic infection. On rectal examination a gland that contains calculi feels hard and irregular and crepitus may be elicited. Prostatic calculi are radio-opaque and therefore visible in X-rays.

Prostatic stones can be removed by transurethral or suprapubic routes, or (if there is benign prostatic hypertrophy) at the time of prostatectomy.

SEMINAL VESICLES

Tuberculosis

Infection of the seminal vesicles is usually tuberculous and the epididymis or the prostate, or both, are usually also involved. Few, if any, symptoms are caused by seminal vesiculitis, and the diagnosis is made after finding tuberculous infection elsewhere in the urinary or genital tract, by feeling the enlarged vesicle on rectal examination, or by detecting calcification of the vesicles in an X-ray of the pelvis.

Carcinoma of the seminal vesicles

The seminal vesicle may be invaded by the spread of carcinoma from the prostate or bladder but is rarely the site of a primary tumour.

THE URETHRA

Infections

Gonorrhoea

This is a venereal infection of the mucous membranes of the genito-urinary tract of both sexes, characterized by a rapidly progressive inflammation of the mucosa of the anterior urethra with a purulent urethral discharge, which contains large numbers of

the diplococcoid Gram-negative gonococcus. The external
urethral meatus may be red and oedematous and balanitis can
occur. If the infection extends into the posterior urethra and
involves the bladder neck, prostate and epididymis, the symptoms
and signs become those of acute prostatitis and epididymitis. If
the infection becomes chronic, urethral sinuses and fistulae and
strictures may develop.

Non-specific urethritis

Non-specific urethritis is any urethritis, in which the
gonococcus can not be found. It can be divided into two
categories. In the first are abacterial urethritis, Reiter's syndrome
and the acute muco—cutaneous syndromes, which are all venereal. In the second category are all the types of urethritis that
are secondary to a variety of pathological and traumatic lesions
and are not venereal.

Abacterial urethritis. The acute form has the same symptoms
and signs as gonorrhoea but the discharge does not contain
gonococci. The subacute form may develop primarily or follow
the acute stage, and can spread to the prostate and epididymis.
The discharge is serous and free of gonococci.

Reiter's syndrome is primary abacterial urethritis associated
with bilateral conjunctivitis and polyarthritis and found only in
males.

Oculomucocutaneous syndromes are abacterial urethritis
associated with such lesions as stomatitis, balanitis, conjunctivitis, arthritis, diarrhoea and a variety of skin lesions.

Traumatic urethritis is the commonest non-venereal cause of
urethritis. The injury may be caused by an indwelling catheter,
endoscopic instruments, external trauma, the use of irritative
chemicals, which may be inserted into the urethra or just used for
washing, or the use of strong contraceptive creams. At first the
urethral discharge contains only the bacterial flora of the normal
urethra but later coliforms, staphylococci or streptococci may
appear. If untreated the infection may spread into the posterior
urethra, prostate, epididymis and even to the bladder and
kidneys.

Miscellaneous. Urethritis may be secondary to such urethral
lesions as strictures, diverticula or tumours.

Trichomonas. Trichomonas vaginalis is probably not an
important cause of urethritis or prostatitis because it can often be

214

found in the normal urethra and any infection it does cause is superficial because it cannot penetrate the mucous membrane. Although trichomonas does little, if any, harm to man, it can be transmitted by intercourse and be responsible for persistent trichomonal vaginitis in the female.

Urethral Strictures

The male urethra varies in calibre not only from one person to another but also from one part to another. A stricture is defined as an abnormal narrowing of the urethra. Urethral strictures may be congenital or acquired. The congenital urethral strictures are discussed in Chapter 11 and only the acquired ones, which may be traumatic or post-infective, will be discussed here.

Traumatic strictures. The injury may be caused by external trauma, which tends to produce strictures in the membranous and spongy parts of the urethra, or by internal trauma which may be caused by endoscopic procedures, operations, indwelling catheters or strong chemicals, and which tends to produce strictures at the external meatus or bladder neck.

Post-infective strictures. Gonorrhoea, abacterial urethritis and the very rare ulcerative diseases of the urethra, such as tuberculosis and syphillis, may all produce strictures. The more severe the infection, the more likely is stricture formation. Of infective strictures about 70 per cent are in the bulbo-membranous urethra and the remainder in the spongy urethra.

Clinical Features of Strictures

Strictures obstruct the flow of urine from the bladder. At first the patient complains of increased frequency, poor calibre and strength of urinary stream, which may spray, terminal dribbling, and later may develop acute or chronic retention and such other sequalae of obstruction as infection, stones and chronic renal failure. Because the urethra is often infected, epididymitis and peri-urethral abscesses may occur. Rupture of a peri-urethral abscess may cause sinuses or urinary fistulae which open on to the skin of the scrotum or perineum.

215

Treatment

Uncomplicated strictures are treated by bougie dilatation which may have to be continued for the rest of the patient's life. The intervals between dilatations may be as long as a year, but are usually 3 to 6 months.

If the stricture is difficult to manage and has to be dilated at short intervals or if dilatation is frequently followed by infection, operation should be considered. If the stricture is short, excision alone may be sufficient, but if a long segment of urethra is involved a reconstruction operation, such as the Denis Browne operation for hypospadias or one of the many modifications, must be carried out.

If a urethral stricture causes retention, it is normally possible to pass a catheter only after the stricture has been dilated under general anaesthesia. If even this fails, the bladder must be drained supra-pubically.

FURTHER READING

Bruce, Sir John, Walmsley, R. & Ross, J. A. (1964). *Manual of Surgical Anatomy.* pp. 412–415. Edinburgh: Livingstone.
Willis, R. A, (1967). *Pathology of Tumours,* 4th ed., pp. 599–609. London: Butterworths.
Winsbury-White, H. P. (1961). *Textbook of Genito-Urinary Surgery,* 2nd ed., pp. 579–654. Edinburgh: Livingstone.

Chapter 14

RETENTION OF URINE

Retention of urine can be acute or chronic.

In acute retention the patient, previously able to pass urine normally or reasonably well, suddenly finds he is unable to pass any despite a painful and urgent desire to do so. The bladder is distended, tense and tender, but the upper urinary tract is usually normal because back pressure and the other effects of obstruction have had insufficient time to damage it.

In chronic retention, the bladder, which has gradually and progressively distended over a period of weeks or even months, is neither tender nor tense, but is often associated with changes, sometimes marked, in the upper urinary tract. The patient with chronic retention may complain only of frequency and dribbling and be quite unaware that his bladder is distended. To detect a chronically distended bladder by palpation and percussion is by no means always easy in an obese patient, and chronic retention may be confused with acute renal failure. For instance, an obese patient in cardiac failure is treated with diuretics, but passes little, if any, urine. It is assumed that he has retention and a catheter is passed. If urine is not obtained it is further assumed that the catheter is not in the bladder, and the patient may be subjected to repeated attempts at catheterization or, even worse, suprapubic cystostomy by stab or open operation, when all the time the bladder is empty. It is always possible to tell if a catheter lies in the bladder or not even if urine does not emerge from it, by injecting about 50 ml of sterile water or saline through the catheter with a bladder syringe. If the fluid passes easily into the catheter without leaking from the urethra when the plunger of the syringe is depressed and returns easily into the syringe when the plunger is withdrawn, the catheter must lie in the bladder.

Causes of Retention

The force with which the bladder contracts and the resistance in the urethra and bladder neck are so balanced that normally the bladder is emptied completely and quickly whenever urine is passed. Retention occurs if either the force with which the bladder contracts is reduced or the resistance in the bladder neck or urethra is increased by obstruction.

The cause of urinary retention may be obvious from the patient's age, history, sex or from the other symptoms and signs associated with it. If the cause is not obvious, efforts should be made to find it, but not too much time should be spent in doing so before relieving a distressed patient of retention.

Neurological

The bladder is supplied by the second, third and fourth sacral nerves. If it is found that the other structures supplied by these nerves, the perianal skin and the anal sphincters, are working satisfactorily, there can be little, if any, decrease in the force with which the bladder contracts. The sensation of the perianal skin and the tone of the anal sphincters can easily be tested by rectal examination, which is as useful for testing the second, third and fourth sacral nerves as it is for examining the prostate. However, most patients with neurological disturbances of the bladder have other signs and symptoms of nervous disease or injuries.

If the cause of retention is not neurological it must be obstructive.

Obstruction

In children obstructive lesions are usually congenital ones in the urethra or bladder neck (p. 188) and can be recognized only by endoscopy or X-ray cystography, but phimosis or a stricture of the external urethral meatus sometimes causes retention and can be recognized by inspection. Urinary retention in children is nearly always chronic and is sometimes associated with such severe changes in the upper urinary tract that a prolonged period of drainage by cystostomy or even ureterostomy is necessary before the obstructive lesion itself can be treated.

In women, obstructive lesions are usually gynaecological such as a subcervical fibroid or a retroverted gravid uterus, and only by vaginal examination, often carried out under general anaesthesia, can they be diagnosed.

In men, obstruction is caused by urethral strictures or prostatic disease. Urethral strictures cause retention at an earlier age than prostatic diseases, but surprisingly few patients with

218

strictures provide a previous history of urethral infection or injury, which are the commonest causes of urethral stricture. Apart from some in the penile urethra, strictures are not palpable and on rectal examination the prostate feels normal. The stricture can be felt on attempting to catheterize the patient, although to pass a catheter into the bladder is usually impossible when stricture is the cause of retention. The stricture should be gently dilated under general anaesthesia and thereafter there should not be any difficulty in passing a catheter. If dilatation fails the bladder must be drained supra-pubically and the stricture treated later.

The prostatic diseases most likely to cause retention are acute infection, chronic infection, benign hypertrophy and carcinoma. Acute prostatic infection rarely causes retention unless it has progressed to abscess formation. The retention, which is associated with marked systemic and local features of infection, should be relieved before the abscess is drained. Although instruments are never passed through an acutely inflamed urethra and rarely through an acutely inflamed prostate, it is reasonable to try to pass a small catheter, but the procedure must be abandoned if the first or second attempt is unsuccessful, and the bladder drained supra-pubically.

In chronic infection, benign hypertrophy or carcinoma, acute retention is relieved by urethral catheterization or, if this fails, by supra-pubic cystostomy; chronic retention need be relieved by catheterization only if it has caused significant chronic renal failure or if the patient is otherwise unwell. In carcinoma, the catheter can be removed some 7 to 10 days after orchidectomy has been done and oestrogen therapy started. If the patient is still unable to pass urine a transurethral resection is carried out. In benign hypertrophy, the later management of the patient is fully discussed on page 207. In chronic infection the catheter may be removed some days after antibiotic therapy has been started but a transurethral resection is usually inevitable if the gland is enlarged or fibrotic enough to cause retention.

Post-operative urinary retention

This may occur after any operation but is most common after abdominal and ano-rectal surgery in the male and after pelvic surgery in the female. The causes are (a) the psychological difficulty of passing urine while confined to bed, (b) flaccidity and weakness of the abdominal wall, (c) undetected obstruction of the urinary tract or damage to the second, third and fourth sacral nerves. Post-operative retention may be avoided by accustoming the patient to the use of a urinal before operation, and by inserting a catheter before operations like abdomino-perineal resection of rectum and pelvic floor repairs, which are inevitably followed by difficulties with micturition.

The muscle fibres of the distended bladder are overstretched and may take several days to recover their tone if the retention is not soon relieved. If the patient is unable to pass urine by sitting or even standing at the side of his bed, a catheter should be passed. Parasympathomimetic drugs like carbachol are best avoided in post-operative patients.

Clot retention

There are two kinds of clot retention. In the first the bladder is distended with urine, but cannot empty because its neck is obstructed by one or more small blood clots. If the patient cannot pass the clot, both clot and urine can usually be evacuated by urethral catheterization. In the second, which may follow operations on the bladder or prostate or severe haemorrhage from tumours of the kidney or bladder, injuries of the kidney or prostatic hypertrophy, the bladder is distended not with urine but with blood and blood clot. The patient is normally shocked not only from the loss of blood but also from viscero-motor reflexes (p. 245) induced by the distended bladder and requires blood transfusion. To evacuate the blood and clot with an ordinary catheter is usually impossible and either a large Tiemann's catheter is used and the bladder washed out with a ground glass syringe (Wardill syringe), or the steel catheter and evacuator designed for washing fragments of stone out of the bladder after lithopaxy. Sometimes even these measures fail and the bladder must be exposed and opened.

Catheterization

Catheterization may damage the urethra or introduce organisms from the environment or from the anterior urethra into the bladder and upper urinary tract, and must be carried out with gentleness and skill. Red rubber catheters are suitable if the catheter is removed as soon as the bladder is empty, but they contain sulphur compounds which may irritate the urethra and if a catheter is to be left in, one made of latex, portex or polyethylene should be used.

For simple catheterization a Jacques catheter can be used, but for prolonged drainage a Foley is preferred which is made of latex and has balloons varying in size from 5 to 100 ml, or a Gibbon catheter, which is a 3-ft long portex tube with two straps, 1 ft from the tip, which are used for securing the catheter to the penis or pubis. A Tiemann catheter has a solid, curved and slightly pointed tip and will often negotiate the elongated prostatic urethra found in many patients with prostatic hypertrophy if other catheters fail. The Harris and whistle-tip catheters are used to drain the bladder after operations on the bladder or prostate.

Supra-pubic Cystostomy

Either a Malecot, a de Pezzer or a Foley catheter may be used to drain the bladder. It can be inserted by open operation or through a trocar and cannula. If retention must be relieved by cystostomy and it is intended to remove the obstructive lesion within a day or two, the bladder may be drained through a large intravenous catheter.

FURTHER READING

Fergusson, J. D. & Williams, J. P. (1969). In *Pye's Surgical Handicraft,* 19th ed., pp. 448–461. Ed. Kyle, J. Bristol: Wright.
McNair, T. J. (1967). *Emergency Surgery,* 8th ed., pp. 792–804. Bristol: Wright.

Chapter 15

DISEASES OF THE TESTES AND EXTERNAL GENITALIA

Anatomy

Testis (Fig. 59)

The testes are ovoid structures loosely attached to the scrotum by the scrotal ligament. Each has a dense fibrous capsule called the tunica albuginea; septa pass from the tunica albuginea into the interior of the testis, and form a fibrous framework for the seminiferous tubules. They end posteriorly in a mass of fibrous

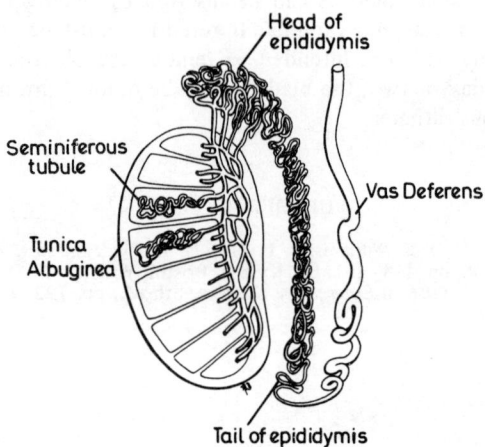

Fig. 59. Anatomy of the testis, epididymis and vas deferens.

tissue called the mediastinum testis. The seminiferous tubules, of which there are about 850 in each testis, are convoluted, but straighten and join each other posteriorly in the mediastinum testis to form a network of short tiny canals called the rete testis. The rete testis becomes the vasa efferentia which perforate the tunica albuginea and carry sperm from the testis into the head of the epididymis. The interstitial, or Leydig, cells lie in the connective tissue between the seminiferous tubules.

Epididymis

Each epididymis is an elongated structure some 5 cm in length applied to the posterior aspect of a testis, and consists of a head, a body and a tail. Sperm pass through its ciliated convoluted canal, from head to tail and on into the vas deferens.

Vas deferens

Each vas deferens is 45 cm long. It begins at the tail of the epididymis and ends by joining the duct of the seminal vesicle to form the ejaculatory duct. In the inguinal canal and scrotum it is loosely bound by connective tissue with its artery, with the testicular artery, with the pampiniform plexus of veins, and with lymphatics and nerves, forming the spermatic cord.

The appendix testis, the appendix epididymis and the paradidymis are vestigial embryonic elements which lie close to the upper pole of the testis and to the epididymis.

Sperm are produced in the testes and matured, protected, nourished and transported by the rest of the genital tract. The interstitial cells of the testis produce testosterone.

Descent of the testes (Fig. 60)

The descent of the testes from the posterior abdominal wall, where they develop, to the scrotum was first described by John Hunter in 1762, but its cause remains a mystery. The testes reach

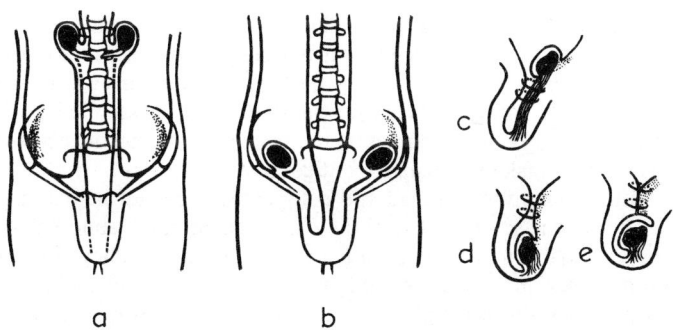

Fig. 60. The descent of the testes.

223

the scrotum before or soon after birth and must be in the scrotum at puberty if spermatogenesis is to take place.

DISEASES OF THE TESTIS

Imperfect Descent of the Testes

A testis which is not in the scrotum may be congenitally absent, which is extremely rare, retractile, ectopic or undescended.

The retractile testis. A retractile testis is one that has been in, or can be manipulated into, the scrotum, but is pulled into an abnormal site, which is usually just outside the external inguinal ring, by spasm of the cremaster muscle. Testes are often retractile during the first two years of life, and occasionally thereafter. At puberty retractile testes invariably descend into the scrotum and treatment is not required for this condition.

Ectopic testis. An ectopic testis is one that has strayed from the normal line of descent during foetal life, and lies in an abnormal site, which is usually the superficial inguinal pouch (which lies between the aponeurosis of the external inguinal ring and the superficial fascia, just lateral to the superficial inguinal ring) and occasionally in the perineum, the femoral canal or the pubo-penile region. An ectopic testis is more normal in size and histology than an incompletely descended one, and its vas deferens and blood vessels are of normal, or near normal, length.

Incompletely descended testis. The incompletely descended testis is one that has been arrested in its normal path of descent and lies in the neck of the scrotum, in the inguinal canal or even in the abdomen. It could be said that the imperfectly descended testis could not make the distance to the scrotum, whereas the ectopic testis could make the distance but got lost on the way.

Incompletely descended and ectopic testes cannot be manipulated into the scrotum, and if they are situated in the abdomen or the inguinal canal they cannot even be palpated. They do not produce sperm, are more liable to torsion, injury and malignant change than normally placed ones, and are often associated with indirect inguinal herniae. They must be treated because only

224

retractile testes descend spontaneously after birth. The incompletely descended or ectopic testis can be most easily diagnosed at birth while it is still under the influence of maternal gonadotrophins, and therefore larger than at any other time before puberty, but most surgeons defer treatment until the child is between 7 and 11 years of age.

Gonadotrophic hormone, which must be given by injection, may hasten the descent of retractile testes, but has no effect on an incompletely descended or ectopic one. Operation is usually inevitable. The incompletely descended or ectopic testis can be mobilized and placed in the scrotum (orchidopexy), or removed (orchidectomy). Unless the testis is in the scrotum at puberty it will never produce sperm and therefore the operation of choice is orchidopexy before puberty, and orchidectomy after puberty. However, if the disease is bilateral orchidopexy should be attempted, even after puberty. The operation of orchidopexy is carried out through an inguinal incision. The testis and cord are thoroughly mobilized and the hernial sac, if any, is excised. The neck of the scrotum, and the scrotum itself, which is usually atrophic, are dilated, the testis is placed in the scrotum and anchored either by temporarily suturing it to the thigh with a silk suture that passes through the scrotum, testis and subcutaneous tissues of the thigh or by placing it in the opposite side of the scrotum (Ombredanne's operation).

Torsion of the Testis

Torsion of the testis (Fig. 61), occurs when the spermatic cord twists at the neck of the scrotum and is sometimes called torsion

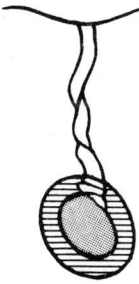

Fig. 61. Torsion of the testis.

225

of the spermatic cord. The twist is usually from without inwards and may be partial or complete. If complete, it varies from one to four turns. Torsion results from the effect of contraction of the cremaster muscle on an abnormally mobile or an inverted testis. A testis will be abnormally mobile if the scrotal ligament, which secures it to the scrotum, is absent, or if the tunica vaginalis invests not only the testis and epididymis but also the lower end of the cord. An inverted testis is one that lies upside down so that the tail of the epididymis and the beginning of the vas lie at the upper pole of the testis.

Torsion deprives the testis of its blood supply. It infarcts, and later atrophies. Injury and exertion are by no means always the cause of torsion, which may even occur during sleep.

Clinical features. When torsion occurs there is severe pain in the testis and iliac fossa, associated with nausea and vomiting, and the scrotum rapidly swells. After 6 to 12 hours gangrene occurs and the pain subsides, but slight fever may develop. To distinguish testis from epididymis by palpation is difficult because both are involved, and because there is usually a blood-stained effusion into the tunica vaginalis and bruising and sometimes oedema of the skin and subcutaneous tissues. The spermatic cord is thickened and sometimes the twist can be palpated. Torsion of the testis is often misdiagnosed as acute epididymitis, but the age of the patient alone should enable a correct diagnosis to be made because epididymitis is uncommon in adolescence when torsion is most frequent.

Treatment. An attempt may be made to undo the twist by manipulation if the patient is seen very soon after the onset of torsion. If manipulation fails, or is not attempted, and provided the patient has been seen within 6 hours of onset, the testis should be explored and the torsion undone. After 6 hours ischaemic changes are irreversible, but orchidectomy need be considered only if severe pain persists. The anomalies that predispose to torsion are usually bilateral, and whatever happens to the twisted testis, the other must be fixed by suturing it to its coverings.

Torsion of an imperfectly descended or ectopic testis is usually indistinguishable from a strangulated inguinal hernia, and should be explored.

Testicular Tumours

Nearly all testicular tumours are malignant and primary and are most commonly found in men between the ages of 20 and 50.

They can be classifed as follows:

1. Seminoma	51 per cent
2. Teratoma	46 per cent
3. Chorionepithelioma	2 per cent
4. Interstitial cell and other tumours	1 per cent.

Seminomas. Seminomas arise from adult cells in the seminiferous tubules. They are homogeneous, cream-coloured tumours, divided into lobules by fibrous septa. Haemorrhage, softening and liquefaction sometimes occur giving the tumour a cystic, variegated appearance.

Teratomas. Teratomas are derived from all three primary germinal layers of the embryo. They vary enormously in their consistence and appearance, and may contain bone, skin, hair follicles and such other tissues. They are usually subdivided into various pathological types, but all are malignant and being embryonic tumours occur at an earlier age than seminomas.

Chorionepitheliomas. Chorionepitheliomas are structurally identical with chorionepithelioma in the female, consisting of trophoblastic tissue with haemorrhage and necrosis.

Most chorionepitheliomas, many teratomas and some seminomas secrete excessive quantities of gonadotrophic hormones which can be detected in the urine by the standard pregnancy tests, and which may cause gynaecomastia.

Spread

Testicular tumours spread, sometimes when the primary is very small, by way of the lymphatics or the blood stream, or both. The lymphatics draining the testis travel along the spermatic cord to the para-aortic glands (not to the inguinal glands), and thence to mediastinal and neck glands. Blood-borne metastases are first found in the lungs and appear in chest X-rays as discrete, spherical opacities in the periphery of the lung fields.

227

Clinical features

Enlargement and hardness of a testis is the first sign of a testicular tumour. On average patients with teratomas wait 6 months and patients with seminomas 12 months after first noticing these features before seeking medical advice. Metastases in glands or lung fields or evidence of excessive gonadotrophic activity will confirm a diagnosis, but this should in any case be easy, because only tumour, syphilis and mumps cause testicular swelling and to exclude syphilis and mumps is not difficult. Nevertheless, one is often misled by thinking that the swelling arises not in the testis but in the coverings of the testis or in the epididymis, and it is then attributed to infection, or haemorrhage. Doubtful scrotal swellings must be explored.

Treatment

Treatment is orchidectomy. The testis is removed together with all its coverings and the spermatic cord, as far as the deep inguinal ring; the cord is clamped or ligated at an early stage of the operation in order to avoid disseminating tumour cells into the veins or lymphatics while mobilizing the testis. Seminomas are sensitive to X-rays and in dealing with them the paravertebral, mediastinal and neck glands are usually irradiated whether or not they appear involved with metastases. Teratomas and chorio-nepitheliomas are radio-resistant and prophylactic radiotherapy is not given, and whether or not metastases should be irradiated is a question requiring separate consideration in each patient. The response of all testicular tumours to antimitotic drugs is unpredictable. Nevertheless, such drugs can be tried in patients who have failed to respond to conventional treatment or have suffered recurrence after it. The drugs recommended are methotrexate, chlorambucil and actinomycin D, but the response of even chorionepitheliomata, which in the female are extremely sensitive to methotrexate, is disappointing.

DISEASES OF THE COVERINGS

Hydrocele

A hydrocele is a collection of straw-coloured fluid within the tunica vaginalis of the testis. The tunica vaginalis is a closed sac derived from the lower part of the processus vaginalis, and has two layers — a visceral, which invests the testis, and a parietal, which lines the internal surface of the scrotum. In the foetus the processus vaginalis precedes the descent of the testis from the abdomen into the scrotum. Its upper part contracts and undergoes obliteration from the deep inguinal ring to within a short distance of the testis, and remains as a thin fibrous cord.

A hydrocele in a normally formed tunica vaginalis is called 'vaginal'. Congenital, infantile and encysted hydroceles occur when the upper part of the processus vaginalis fails to close in whole or in part (Fig. 62).

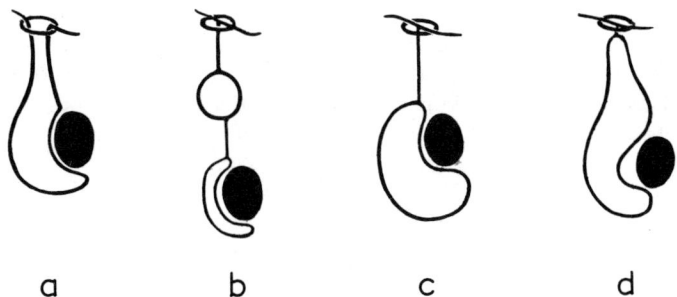

a   b   c   d

Fig. 62. Varieties of hydrocele. a. Congenital. b. Encysted (hydrocele of the cord). c. Vaginal. d. Infantile.

Vaginal hydrocele. The distended tunica forms a pear-shaped swelling which is translucent, and which reaches the external inguinal ring. At first the tunica itself and the testes are unaltered, but later, especially if the hydrocele has been repeatedly aspirated, the tunica undergoes fibrous thickening and may even calcify, and the testis is compressed and atrophies. Some hydroceles are secondary to disease of the testis or epididymis, but only when the fluid has been aspirated can the other contents of the scrotum be palpated. Vaginal hydroceles can be treated by aspirating the fluid and injecting a sclerosant, like quinine urethane, or by excising or everting the hydrocele sac through a scrotal or inguinal incision.

Congenital hydrocele. A congenital hydrocele occurs when all the processus vaginalis remains patent, and communicates with the peritoneal cavity. The accumulation of fluid within the sac may be secondary to ascites or tuberculous peritonitis. The hydrocele fluid disappears inside the abdominal cavity when the scrotum is elevated. The communication between peritoneal cavity and hydrocele is usually too small for a hernia to develop.

Infantile hydrocele. An infantile hydrocele arises when the upper part of the processus vaginalis seals off at the deep inguinal ring, but is not obliterated. The tunica and the upper part of the processus vaginalis distend with fluid as far as the internal inguinal ring, without communicating with the peritoneal cavity.

Encysted hydrocele (hydrocele of the cord). An encysted hydrocele develops when fusion and obliteration of the upper part of the processus vaginalis is incomplete. It forms a smooth oval discrete swelling which is associated with the spermatic cord, and which may be mistaken for an irreducible inguinal hernia.

Haematocele

A haematocele is a collection of blood within the tunica vaginalis and is caused by injury or torsion, and can be treated by aspiration. An old clotted haematocele may be indistinguishable from a testicular neoplasm and should be explored.

CYSTS OF THE EPIDIDYMIS AND SPERMATOCELE

Cysts of the Epididymis

These are more frequently found than spermatoceles. They contain clear fluid and are usually multilocular, translucent, bilateral and situated behind the testis (Fig. 63).

Cysts of the Appendix of the Testis

The appendix of the testis (sometimes called the hydatid of Morgagni) is an embryonic remnant at the upper pole of the testis and is prone to cystic change. The cyst forms a small pedunculated, translucent swelling at the upper pole of the testis and is liable to undergo torsion.

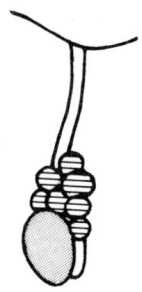

Fig. 63. Cysts of the epididymis.

Spermatocele

A spermatocele is a unilocular cyst derived from some portion of the sperm-conducting system of the epididymis. They are filled with opalescent fluid, and situated in the head of the epididymis above and behind the testis. They can be aspirated or excised, but rarely cause symptoms unless very large (Fig. 64).

EPIDIDYMO-ORCHITIS

Although the word epididymo-orchitis suggests that both testis and epididymis are simultaneously infected, the primary infections of the testis, syphilis and mumps, do not involve the epididymis, and the organisms that primarily infect the epididymis, *E. coli,* enterococci, gonococci, tuberculosis, etc., only

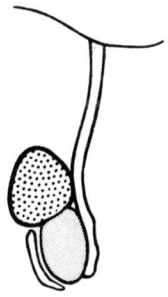

Fig. 64. Spermatocele.

extend into the testis when the disease is advanced. Therefore, there can be either orchitis or epididymitis. To speak of epididymo-orchitis is convenient because it can be very difficult to distinguish the testis from the epididymis in an infected scrotum. Nevertheless, an effort must be made to do so because if the testis alone is involved it can be infected only if the patient has syphilis or mumps.

Orchitis

Only mumps and syphilis primarily infect the testis.

Mumps orchitis. Orchitis, sometimes bilateral, occurs in about 1 out of every 4 males who contract mumps after puberty. It usually develops about a week after the onset of the disease, when the affected salivary glands are resolving. It begins with fever, rigors, vomiting and swelling of the testis, which may not be very painful. Resolution begins within 3 to 4 days, but atrophy, which may not be obvious for 1½ to 2 years, occurs in about 50 per cent of patients.

Syphilitic orchitis. Syphilitic orchitis is rare, and of its various forms only two will be mentioned.

Latent syphilis. In this condition large numbers of spirochaetes appear in the seminal fluid, although the testis may appear normal on clinical examination.

Gumma. Gumma is a late manifestation of tertiary syphilis and sometimes bilateral. It presents as a space-occupying lesion in the testis indistinguishable from tumour. If one is in doubt about the diagnosis it is better to remove a disorganized syphilitic testis than to miss a testicular tumour.

Epididymitis

Acute

Many micro-organisms including *E. coli,* enterococci, staphylococci, gonococci and tuberculosis can infect the epididymis, which they reach either by the blood stream or along the vas deferens from the posterior urethra, or prostate. The acute phase consists of a 'flu-like illness' with malaise, fever and often rigors followed by or associated with pain, redness, swelling and

232

tenderness in the scrotum. A secondary hydrocele may develop and increase the difficulty of distinguishing epididymis from testis. Most cases subside with rest and antibiotics, but sometimes an abscess forms and has to be drained.

Chronic

This may be caused by tubercle bacillus or *E. coli.*

Genital tuberculosis

This is always secondary to tuberculosis elsewhere and in 50 per cent of cases is associated with tuberculosis of the urinary tract. The prostate, the seminal vesicles and the epididymis are involved separately or together. Tuberculosis of the prostate and seminal vesicles is asymptomatic in its early stages, and attention is usually first drawn to the disease when, and if, epididymitis develops. Tuberculosis epididymitis may begin acutely and be indistinguishable from non-specific infections, but is usually insidious. The epididymis enlarges and becomes hard, craggy, but is only slightly tender. The vas deferens may be elongated or beaded. Later the epididymis becomes fixed to the skin of the scrotum and a sinus may form. Secondary hydroceles are uncommon, and on rectal examination it may be found that the prostate or the seminal vesicles, or both, are involved. The body of the testis remains uninvolved in more than 80 per cent of cases.

Treatment. Genital tuberculosis is treated with antituberculous chemotherapy and operation is rarely necessary. However, if the diagnosis is in doubt, exploration should be carried out at an early date because it is safer to explore a tuberculosis epididymis than to give antituberculous chemotherapy for a testicular tumour.

DISEASES OF THE PAMPINIFORM PLEXUS

Varicocele

A varicocele is a varicose condition of the veins of the spermatic cord which become dilated, elongated and tortuous (Fig. 65). Some left-sided varicoceles are secondary to thrombosis or tumour in the left renal vein (into which the left testicular vein drains), and unlike idiopathic ones do not empty when the scrotum is elevated.

only be possible after a dorsal slit has been made in the prepuce. Circumcision should be carried out later.

Carcinoma of the penis

Carcinoma of the penis is rarely seen before the age of 50, and is never seen in people who have been circumcised in infancy. It is usually associated with phimosis, balanitis and chronic irritation. The tumour is a squamous cell carcinoma which may be proliferative or ulcerative. It usually occurs on the glans or on the inside of the prepuce. It is often hidden by the prepuce and obscured by secondary balanitis. The disease is usually of low malignancy but may spread down the shaft of the penis and to the inguinal lymph glands. It can be treated either by radiotherapy or by surgery, and is sometimes so localized that a partial resection is curative.

Injuries

Avulsion of penile skin, or even the whole penis, may occur with severe trauma.

Annular constriction. Ligatures or rings of various sorts, which are usually self-applied, produce annular constriction and may cause ischaemia and gangrene.

Rupture of the corpora cavernosa. The corpora cavernosa may be ruptured or displaced from the pubis in injuries of the erected penis.

All severe penile injuries may be associated with injury to the urethra and extravasation of urine.

SCROTUM

Cellulitis

Cellulitis of the scrotum may occur spontaneously or result from injury. It is associated with extensive oedema because the tissues are loose, and sometimes with gangrene, particularly if the organism is a haemolytic streptococcus.

Carcinoma of the scrotum

Carcinoma of the scrotum was recognized as an occupational disease by Pott in 1775, who called it 'chimney-sweep's cancer'. Later it was called 'mule-spinner's cancer'. The tumour is a squamous cell carcinoma of low malignancy and slow growth,

236

which begins as a proliferative lesion and later ulcerates. It may spread by the lymphatics to the inguinal lymph nodes.

FURTHER READING

Brown, J. J. M. (1962). *Surgery of Childhood.* pp. 1135–1181. London: Arnold.
Willis, R. A. (1967). *Pathology of Tumours,* 4th ed., pp. 568–597. London: Butterworths.
Winsbury-White, H. P. (1961). *Textbook of Genito-Urinary Surgery,* 2nd ed., pp. 646–668. Edinburgh: Livingstone.

Chapter 16

NEUROLOGICAL DISTURBANCES OF BLADDER FUNCTION

PHYSIOLOGY OF MICTURITION

Micturition, or the act of passing urine, involves the bladder and the urethra, and the visceral and somatic nervous reflexes which, under the influence of higher centres, control their activity. Normal micturition is so efficient that it does not start until we experience and decide not to suppress the desire to pass urine, but once started, it continues until the bladder is empty.

Anatomy

The smooth muscle fibres of the bladder are reticulate, except around the neck of the bladder where they are spiral or longitudinal, and continue down the urethra as far as the external sphincter. The reticulate muscle fibres of the bladder are collectively called the detrusor muscle. In males the external sphincter is a separate striated muscle that surrounds the membranous part of the urethra. In females external sphincteric action is carried out, not by a separate muscle as in males but by the anterior part of the levator ani.

Contraction of the smooth muscle of the bladder, bladder neck and urethra is initiated by parasympathetic fibres from the second, third and fourth sacral segments, and inhibited by sympathetic fibres from the coeliac, hypogastric, inferior mesenteric and aortic plexuses, which pass to the bladder through the presacral nerve. However, sympathetic activity plays little, if any, part in normal micturition. Contraction of the external sphincter, or in females the anterior part of the levator ani, is initiated by the pudendal nerve, also from the second, third and fourth sacral segments. Afferent fibres from the bladder and posterior urethra enter the second, third and fourth sacral segments of the spinal cord (which may be regarded as the spinal

238

centre for micturition). Those from the bladder travel alongside the parasympathetic nerves, those from the urethra in the pudendal nerve. The spinal centre for micturition is connected with higher centres by both ascending and descending tracts (Fig. 66).

Except during micturition, the urethra is closed and empty of urine. It is kept closed by the numerous elastic fibres interposed between the smooth muscle fibres in its wall, assisted by the tonic contraction of the external sphincter which can be increased by voluntary effort. However, the elastic fibres alone are capable of keeping the urethra closed. During micturition, contraction of the smooth muscle in the bladder neck and urethra opens the bladder neck and opens and shortens the urethra because the muscle fibres are longitudinally disposed. Contrary to popular belief, in the resting state the urethra is closed. To open it requires the work of muscular contraction.

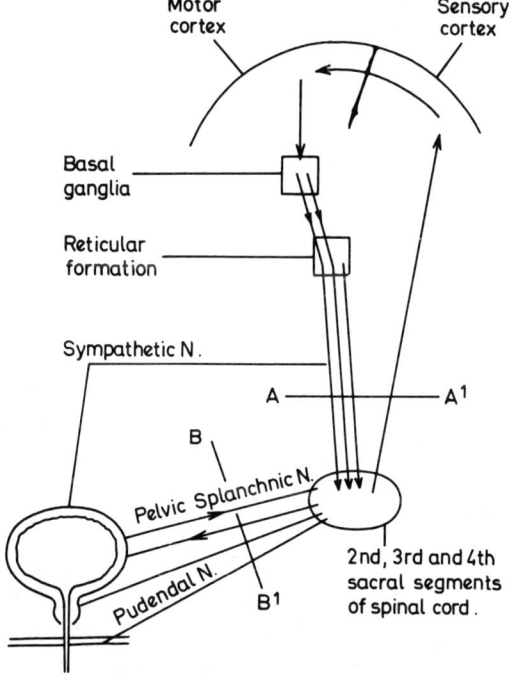

Fig. 66. Shows the nerves supplying the bladder and the urethra, and their connections with the sensory cortex and the higher motor centres.

Physiology

As the bladder fills, the spinal centre for micturition receives more excitor impulses from the stretch receptors in the bladder wall, and at the same time, more and more inhibitory impulses from the higher motor centres (the cortex, the basal ganglia and the reticular formation). The central excitatory state of the spinal centre hardly changes until the bladder contains 300 or 400 ml of urine when it increases and impulses then pass to the sensory cortex and produce the desire to pass urine. If it is inconvenient to pass urine the higher motor centres increase their inhibitory influence on the spinal centre and the desire fades. If it is convenient to pass urine the inhibitory influence of the higher motor centres is removed and the spinal centre becomes excited enough to send impulses along the parasympathetic nerves and contracts the smooth muscle of the bladder, the bladder neck and the urethra. Urine enters the posterior urethra. Pudendal afferent nerves are stimulated and inhibit the anterior horn cells of the pudendal efferent nerve. The external sphincter relaxes and urine passes through the urethra and external urethral meatus. The higher motor centres, which inhibit the spinal centre for micturition while the bladder fills, bombard it with facilitatory impulses once micturition starts and so keep the bladder contracting until it is empty.

Components of Micturition

Micturition may be divided into the following components:

Sensation. The bladder is generously supplied with stretch, touch, pain and temperature sensory endings but only the stretch receptors are of importance in micturition. They are stimulated as the bladder fills and the impulses, which travel to the spinal centre for micturition and thence in the lateral spinothalamic tract to the cortex, are responsible for the desire to pass urine.

Capacity. The normal bladder capacity is defined, not as the amount of urine the bladder can hold, but as the amount of urine the bladder contains when we experience a strong desire to pass urine. It varies between 300 and 400 ml. It is reduced, sometimes considerably, if the higher motor centres do not inhibit the spinal centre as the bladder fills.

240

Uninhibited contraction. Micturition is under voluntary control and begins only when we wish it to do so. The desire to pass urine can be suppressed if we experience it at an inconvenient time. Uninhibited contractions occur only if the higher motor centres do not inhibit the spinal centre.

Residual urine. With normal micturition, the bladder is completely emptied and there is no residual urine. The bladder may fail to empty if the higher centres do not facilitate the spinal centre during micturition or if there is obstruction.

Bladder tone. The pressure inside the normal bladder varies between 1 and 4 cm/water when empty, and 4 and 15 cm/water when full. The bladder is able to accommodate increasing quantities of urine with little, if any, increase in pressure because, as it fills, it progressively relaxes. This relaxation is partly the effect of neuromuscular activity (inhibitory influence of higher motor centres) and partly the result of rheological properties which the bladder, like all muscle, possesses by virtue of its high viscosity.

Cystometry

The bladder can be studied by introducing varying volumes of fluid into it and recording the pressure they produce. The procedure is carried out by introducing a 2-way catheter into the bladder. The bladder is emptied and the amount of residual urine, if any, is measured. One limb of the catheter is connected to a reservoir of sterile fluid and the other to a recording manometer (Figs. 67 and 68).

Cystometry is a useful investigation but as much about a patient's bladder function can often be discovered by taking a careful history and carrying out a physical examination. A patient who needs to pass urine when the bladder contains some 300 or 400 ml, who can suppress the need, who is continent, and who empties the bladder completely when micturition occurs, has normal bladder function.

NEUROLOGICAL DISTURBANCES OF BLADDER FUNCTION

The function of the bladder can be disordered in various ways when its nerve supply is damaged by injury or disease.

241

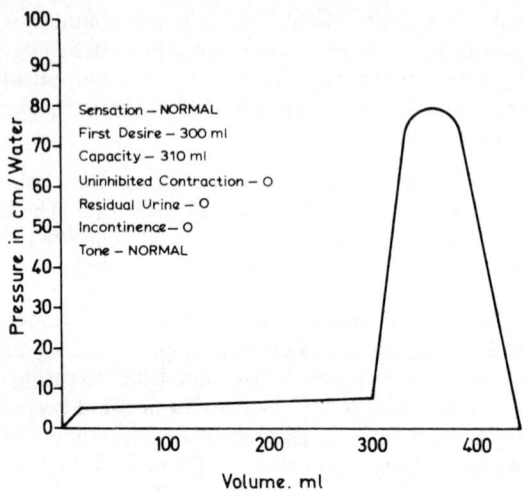

Fig. 67. The features and a typical cystometrogram of the normal bladder.

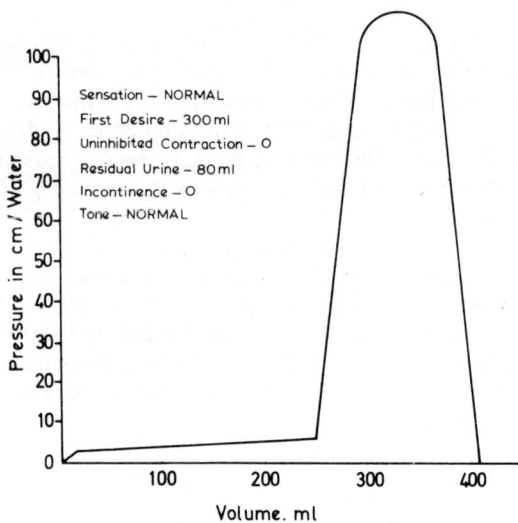

Fig. 68. The features and a typical cystometrogram of a bladder that has hypertrophied because of prostatic obstruction. Despite the very powerful and sustained contraction, the residual urine, which was estimated before the tracing was started, is 85 ml.

242

Uninhibited Bladder

If the higher motor centres do not inhibit or, worse, facilitate the spinal centre as the bladder fills, uninhibited micturition occurs (Fig. 69). The need to pass urine is experienced when the bladder contains as little as 50 or 100 ml of urine, and because it cannot be suppressed the patient complains of frequency and urgency and of the urge incontinence during the day and of enuresis at night. However, as there is nothing wrong with facilitation, micturition continues until the bladder is empty, and since there is no residual urine there is no more risk of infection, stones and renal failure than with normal micturition. Normal bladders often behave as uninhibited ones in cold weather or at times of nervous tension or anxiety, when lower motor neurones are facilitated by the reticular formation. Persistent uninhibited micturition is caused by psychological disturbances and may respond to the appropriate treatment assisted by the use of smooth muscle relaxants, like Pro-Banthine, Cetiprin or Buscopan.

The Atonic Bladder

The atonic bladder causes no desire to pass urine, cannot contract even tonically and is distended by a large volume of residual urine which overflows in small quantities at frequent intervals through the urethra (Fig. 70). It causes back pressure and predisposes to infection, stones and vesico-ureteric reflux. The smooth muscle fibres of the bladder are overstretched and may be permanently damaged.

The bladder becomes atonic in two circumstances: (1) during the period of spinal shock that follows sudden separation of the spinal cord or cauda equina from the higher centres by trauma or acute infection. After spinal shock wears off, which lasts about 6 weeks in humans, the bladder becomes automatic or autonomous depending on the level of the lesion. (2) In chronic diseases, such as diabetic neuropathy and tabes dorsalis, when the sensory pathways from the bladder are diseased, but the motor pathways remain intact. If both motor and sensory pathways, or motor alone, are involved, the bladder becomes automatic or autonomous.

Attempts can be made to empty the atonic bladder by

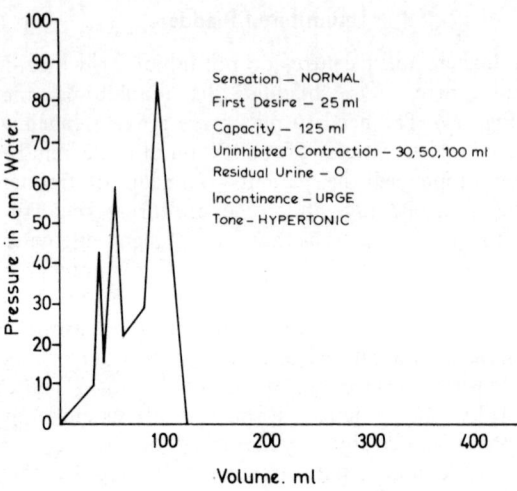

Fig. 69. The features and a typical cystometrogram of an uninhibited bladder.

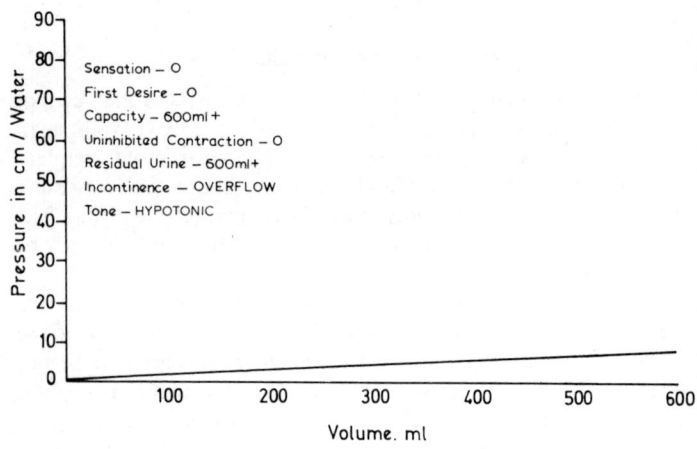

Fig. 70. The features and a typical cystometrogram of an atonic bladder.

stimulating it with parasympathomimetic drugs like carbachol, by reducing the resistance at the bladder neck with a transurethral resection, by manual compression, which can be dangerous because more urine may pass up the ureter than through the urethra, or by draining the bladder with a urethral or supra-pubic

244

catheter. During the period of spinal shock the atonic bladder should be kept empty with an indwelling urethral catheter. The permanent atonic bladder of patients with tabes dorsalis or diabetic neuropathy may have to be permanently drained with a urethral or supra-pubic catheter, or excluded by diverting urine to the skin. Urine must never be diverted into the colon in patients with some neurological disturbance of the bladder because the rectum and anus are supplied by the same nerve roots as the bladder and urine will leak from the anus, leaving the patient worse off than before.

Automatic Bladder (Upper Motor Neurone Bladder)

The bladder becomes an automatic one following a complete, or nearly complete, section of the spinal cord above the sacral centre for micturition after the period of spinal shock is over (Fig. 71). Because sensory impulses cannot reach the cerebral cortex, there is no desire to micturate, and because inhibitory impulses cannot reach the spinal centre, the bladder is hypertonic, its capacity is reduced and it contracts automatically when it contains 200 to 250 ml of urine. Because facilitatory impulses cannot reach the sacral centre, however, the bladder does not contract strongly enough or long enough to empty completely and there is residual urine.

Autonomous Bladder (Lower Motor Neurone Bladder)

The bladder becomes autonomous with a complete, or nearly complete, transection of the spinal cord below the second, third and fourth sacral segments, or of the cauda equina, or of the second, third and fourth sacral nerves. Because sensory impulses cannot reach the cerebral cortex there is no desire to micturate, and because inhibitory impulses cannot reach the bladder it is hypertonic and its capacity is reduced. The bladder does contract but its contractions are weak and inco-ordinate. Little urine is passed and the amount of residual urine is high (Fig. 72).

In both the automatic and autonomous types of bladder, viscero-motor and viscero-sensory reflexes may be exaggerated and cause sweating, changes in skin colour and increased blood pressure as the bladder fills.

245

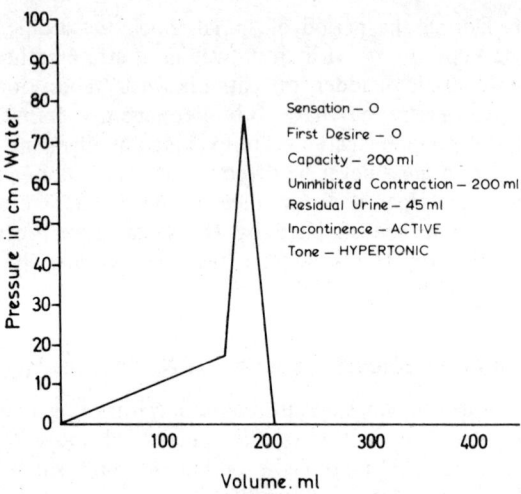

Fig. 71. The features and a typical cystometrogram of an automatic bladder.

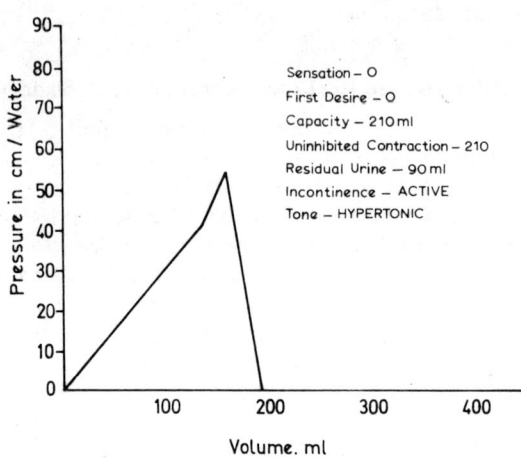

Fig. 72. The features and a typical cystometrogram of an autonomous bladder.

246

Voluntary Neurogenic Bladder

This phase, contradictory as it may be, is a useful description of such disturbances of micturition as may occur with incomplete lesions of the nerve supply of the bladder. Because the nerves to the bladder are bilaterally represented and overlap, many incomplete lesions, including hemisection of the cord or complete division of all the nerves on one or other side, do not always disturb micturition. If they do, some sensation of bladder filling always remains and considerable improvement in bladder function can be expected, provided the nervous lesion is not a progressive one. Two types of bladder behaviour may result from partial lesions:

1. If both inhibitory and facilitatory pathways to the spinal centre are defective, the bladder capacity is reduced, sensation is retained, but the desire to pass urine cannot be suppressed. The bladder does not empty completely and there is residual urine. The patient complains of urgency, urge incontinence and sometimes enuresis. This disturbance causes symptoms identical with those of the uninhibited bladder, with which it is often confused, but unlike the uninhibited bladder it is associated with residual urine and therefore predisposes to infection, stones and chronic renal failure.

2. If facilitation alone is defective, the bladder is hypotonic and has a large capacity. Some sensation of filling is retained, but the bladder does not contract well enough to empty and there is residual urine and sometimes overflow incontinence. This bladder disturbance results not only from neurological disturbance but also from the damage muscle fibres of the bladder suffer if they have been overstretched for a prolonged time. They may recover if the bladder is drained with a urethral catheter for some time.

Treatment

The aim is to train patients who have neurological disease to make the best possible use of what bladder function remains because normal bladder function cannot be restored unless the lesion is temporary, or nerve fibres regenerate. Useful as classifications of bladder dysfunction may be, only two things need to be known about micturition in order to manage the patient.

The two main problems are, firstly, residual urine which predisposes to infection, stones, back pressure and chronic renal failure, and secondly, incontinence. Patients should be encouraged to micturate at regular intervals by the clock, and to assist bladder emptying by tapping the abdominal wall or by moderate manual compression. Some patients can recognize bladder filling by manifestations of exaggerated viscero-sensory or viscero-motor reflexes such as sweating, changes in skin colour, headache and palpitations. The bladder may be stimulated with parasympatho-mimetic drugs, infection and stones may be prevented not only by reducing residual urine to a minimum, but also by encouraging a high fluid intake, by treating any infection detected by routine examination of the urine, by encouraging mobility, and by excluding excessive quantities of calcium-rich foods from the diet. The immobility of paraplegia not only predisposes to pressure sores, but also hinders drainage of urine from the renal pelves and causes decalcification of bones.

Many patients with neurological disturbances of bladder function develop secondary obstruction to the outflow of urine from the bladder. If the amount of residual urine increases or fails from the beginning to reach acceptable levels, obstruction must be looked for at the bladder neck or at the external sphincter. At the bladder neck, obstruction can be treated by a transurethral resection, at the external sphincter, by injecting or dividing the pudendal nerves.

The life expectancy of the paraplegic or quadraplegic patient depends upon his attaining and maintaining a low volume of residual urine and thereby avoiding such sequelae as infections, stones, back pressure and chronic renal failure. Incontinence is very inconvenient but unlike residual urine it does not reduce life expectancy. Although it is often improved by the measures used to reduce the volume of residual urine, many patients have to wear a portable urinal. In women incontinence, if severe and disabling, may demand permanent drainage of the bladder with an indwelling catheter or diversion of the urine to the skin, because they cannot be satisfactorily fitted with an appliance.

Enuresis

Enuresis or bed-wetting is the involuntary escape of urine during sleep. It is abnormal after the age of 3 years, by which time most children have normal urinary and anal control and normal habits of micturition and defaecation.

About 10 per cent of patients who present with enuresis have organic disease in the urinary tract or nervous system, but most, if not all, of these patients have symptoms and signs other than enuresis, which make it possible, if not to diagnose the lesion, at least to recognize the need for further investigation of the urinary tract or nervous system. In the urinary tract the lesion is usually one that obstructs the outflow of urine from the bladder like congenital strictures of the urethra or bladder neck, urethral valves or phimosis, but patients with infection, stones, ectopic ureters or other abnormalities may complain of enuresis. In the nervous system myelomeningocele, transverse myelitis and injuries may cause enuresis but invariably manifest other features of neurological abnormality.

In the remaining 90 per cent, no organic disease is found in the urinary tract or nervous system, but some, about 20 per cent, have uninhibited bladders and may also complain of frequency, urgency and urge incontinence during the day. In all these patients the cause is defective training or psychological factors or a combination of each. Many have a spina bifida occulta, but it is unlikely to be an aetiological factor because less than 5 per cent of patients with this anomaly have any neurological abnormality. There is no reliable cure for enuresis and treatment is based upon training the patient to acquire regular habits of micturition and defaecation. The fluid intake can be restricted after 5 or 6 p.m. A child can be wakened during the night and encouraged to pass urine. Drugs to lighten sleep, like ephedrine, or to relax the bladder, like Pro-Banthine, can be tried. Many alarm devices have been designed. All waken the child when his voided urine closes an electric circuit and rings a bell or delivers an electric shock. Older patients may be trained to waken themselves with an alarm clock which is set to ring just before the suspected time of bed wetting, but it is surprising how many enuretics are reluctant to do much to help themselves.

FURTHER READING

Bell, G. H., Davidson, J. N. & Scarborough, H. (1968). *Textbook of Physiology and Biochemistry,* 7th ed., pp. 729–733. Edinburgh: Livingstone.
Eckstein, H. B. (1968). In *Paediatric Urology,* pp. 365–387. Ed. Williams, D. I. London: Butterworths.
Riches, Sir Eric (1970). *Modern Trends in Urology* – 3, pp. 312–337. London: Butterworths.

Chapter 17

INFERTILITY IN THE MALE

Conception can occur only if normal spermatozoa contact the ovum during its passage from fallopian tubes to uterus. The male not only contributes spermatozoa but is also responsible for placing them in the upper vagina whence they can easily travel through the cervix into the uterus. In all cases of sterility both male and female partners must be examined. The husband should be examined first because elaborate tests are needed to establish fertility in the female whereas quite simple ones will do so in the male. How many wives of sterile husbands have needlessly endured a long series of investigations and even treatments, when all could have been avoided had the husband been examined first.

In the male fertility depends on three factors: (1) intercourse, (2) ejaculation and (3) the quality of the seminal fluid.

Intercourse

Inability to have intercourse is called impotence. It may be the result of penile abnormalities, like hypospadias or of nervous disorders, like paraplegia or diabetic neuropathy, but is usually psychological and found in men who are otherwise physically normal.

Ejaculation

Obviously ejaculation does not occur in men who are impotent. Ejaculation may also not occur, even though intercourse is satisfactory, in men who have had operations on the bladder neck or prostate because the ejaculate passes retrogradely into the bladder, or in those who have urethral strictures.

Seminal fluid

The normal volume of the ejaculate is between 2 and 3 ml. Only 5 per cent is spermatozoa, the rest is secretion from the prostate and seminal vesicles. A normal ejaculate contains more, often considerably more, than 40,000,000 spermatozoa per ml, and of these at least 50 per cent are motile and no more than 40 per cent abnormal forms. An absence of sperm is called azoospermia, a reduced number oligospermia.

If intercourse is satisfactory and the seminal fluid normal the patient's fertility is regarded as normal.

If the patient is oligospermic or azoospermic a careful history must be taken and a physical examination carried out. In the history particular attention should be paid to diseases or operations that may involve the testes or sperm-conducting systems, such as mumps, injuries, undescended testes, operations on testes or inguinal areas, urethritis or epididymitis. In examining the patient an assessment is made of the size and consistence of the testes, the state of the vas and epididymis and the presence of varicoceles. Fertility has little, if any, relationship to general physical development.

Treatment

Oligospermia

If the patient has a varicocele, it should be treated, preferably by high ligation. Ligation of a varicocele in an oligospermic patient often improves the quality of the seminal fluid.

Otherwise an attempt may be made to stimulate spermatogenesis with androgens, human gonadotrophins or clomiphene citrate. There is evidence that complete spermatogenesis depends on androgens as well as on follicle-stimulating hormone, but the response of oligospermia to androgens and to gonadotrophins, which are very expensive and have to be injected, is unpredictable. Clomiphene citrate, an analogue of chlorotrianisene, increases the urinary excretion of follicle-stimulating hormone and of 17–ketosteroid. The mechanism of its action has not yet been clarified but it has been shown to improve the seminal fluid in some oligospermic patients.

Azoospermia

If the testes are soft and atrophic or undescended it may be concluded that spermatogenesis is not taking place and that the azoospermia is irreversible.

If the testes appear normal in size and consistence a testicular biopsy should be carried out. If this reveals defective spermato-genesis an attempt can be made to stimulate the testes with the same drugs used in oligospermia. If it reveals normal spermato-genesis it is concluded that there must be an obstruction in the sperm-conducting mechanism. Such an obstruction is usually at or near the tail of the epididymis and can be short-circuited by the operation of vaso-epididymostomy in which the vas is anas-tomosed beyond the obstructed segment to the head of the epididymis.

Almost as much study, but far less publicity, has been devoted to the problems of infertility as to the problems of birth control. Knowledge of the mechanisms involved in sperm production, morphology and transport has greatly increased, but less progress has been made in treatment and many infertile couples must content themselves with adoption.

FURTHER READING

Hanley, H. G. (1960). Infertility in men. *Practitioner,* **185,** 137–143.
Hotchkiss, R. S. (1963). In *Urology,* 2nd ed., Vol. I, pp. 643–680. Ed. Campbell, M. F. Philadelphia: Saunders.

INDEX

Printed by R. & R. Clark Ltd, Edinburgh